Past Imperfect

How tracing your family medical history can save your life

Past Imperfect

How tracing your family medical history can save your life

Carol Daus

Foreword by Jeanne Homer, M.S.
Genetic Counselor

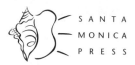

SANTA
MONICA
PRESS

© 1999 SANTA MONICA PRESS LLC
P.O. Box 1076
Santa Monica, CA 90406
1-800-784-9553
www.santamonicapress.com

Printed in the United States

Santa Monica Press books are available at special quantity discounts
when purchased in bulk by corporations, organizations, or groups.
Please call our Special Sales department at 1-800-784-9553.

*This book is intended to provide general information. It is not intended to
replace the advice of your physician or medical counselor. The publisher,
author, distributor, and copyright owner are not engaged in rendering health,
medical, or other professional advice or services, and are not liable or responsible to any person or group with respect to any loss, illness, or injury caused
or alleged to be caused by the information found in this book.*

Library of Congress Cataloging-in-Publication Data

Daus, Carol, 1958-
Past imperfect : how tracing your family medical history can
save your life / by Carol Daus, Jeanne Homer.
p.   cm.
Includes bibliographical references.
ISBN 1-891661-03-5
1. Medical genetics. 2. Genealogy. 3. Medical records. [ ] I.
Homer, Jeanne. II. Title.
RB155 .D35 1999
616'.042—dc21   98-32131
                                                 CIP

10 9 8 7 6 5 4 3 2 1

Book and cover design by Ad Infinitum
Cover hand image © 1999 PhotoDisc, Inc.

Contents

Foreword

If unearthing your family medical history only made you aware of your ultimate fate, it would have limited value. The reality is that discovering your medical history can make a difference in your future. Many disorders have a genetic component, over which you have no control, as well as an "environmental" element, in which you do have a say. In other words, lifestyle can shift the scales and determine whether or not a genetic propensity toward a disease will become a reality. And in illnesses where heredity plays a larger role, awareness and early detection can have an enormous impact on the outcome.

At the very least, if you research your family medical history, you will become aware of some potential problems and can prepare yourself to deal with them. As a prenatal genetic counselor, I see many couples with a family history of multiple miscarriages. If you have a similar history, you may have a 1 in 20 chance of having a child with birth defects and mental retardation. A blood test can tell you if you are at an increased risk, and if you are, then you may want to have genetic testing during your pregnancy or choose other options for having children.

Past Imperfect is a step-by-step guide to the ins and outs of tracing your family medical history. Carol Daus's expert advice ranges from hints on how to broach this potentially sensitive subject with your relatives to what information can be gleaned from cemeteries! *Past Imperfect* has the unusual distinction of being not only an excellent reference manual on both genetics and genealogy, but it is also a book that is interesting and enjoyable to sit down and read from start to finish. Her examples of real-life families poignantly illustrate the value of undertaking this pursuit. She then does much of the legwork for you, by providing myriad phone numbers, addresses, and even websites in the appendices. There is also a superb compendium of common genetic disorders, including a wealth of information on inheritance, treatment, and prevention.

Following are examples of how *Past Imperfect* can play a significant role in not only your health, but the health of your entire family:

- If realizing that adult-onset diabetes runs in your family gives you the incentive to improve your diet and adopt an exercise program, then these actions may delay the onset of the disease or prevent it altogether!

- Twenty-five to fifty percent of patients with bipolar disorder (manic depression) attempt suicide once, and 19% of manic-depressive patients die due to suicide. The peak age of onset of this illness is in the 15–19 age range. So, if you discover that your relatives suffer from this disorder, keep a close eye on your teenagers and don't delay in getting treatment at the first signs.

- Response to medications can also be an inherited tendency. For instance, if depression runs in your family and it took five attempts to get the correct prescription that finally helped your mother, find out which medications had unpleasant side effects and which one did the trick.

- Alternatively, you may be reassured that you have escaped the malady present in your ancestors based on the inheritance pattern of the disease. A patient of mine whose uncle had suffered from hemophilia was relieved to know that his own children were no more at risk than mine to be born with this potentially serious ailment.

Every week we are discovering the locations of a growing number of genes, new tests are being developed, and we are solving the mysteries of inherited diseases. Genetic information can be very complex, and the issues surrounding inherited disorders can often be clouded by questions of guilt, blame, and simply incorrect information. Nearly every day, I listen to how my patients have dealt with the imperfect past of their families: One mother informed me that her daughter's thalassemia was from "the other side of the family." (Thalassemia, in fact, is always inherited from both the mother and the father.) Again and again I hear that a niece or nephew was born with a cleft lip or a heart defect because "his father used drugs in the '70s" (not a possible cause of these conditions).

Another of my patients told me recently that he was not concerned about a strong family history of manic depression because, "it only affects the women in my family." (Actually, that was by chance, since manic depression affects males and females equally.) And then there was the expectant father who was mildly affected with type 1 neurofibromatosis who was not aware that, even within the same family, this disease, for unknown reasons, can strike some members very severely, even causing cancer, while others escape with only freckles in the armpit region. Each of his children faces 50-50 odds of inheriting the faulty gene from him.

For these reasons, if you have any questions or concerns, as *Past Imperfect* states so clearly, it's important to meet with your doctor or a genetics professional. He or she will analyze your family tree and then provide an individualized risk assessment for you and your children. Genetic testing may be offered, or referrals or recommendations will be tailored to your specific needs.

And now, Carol Daus will be your guide as you embark on an adventure that will, at the least, be fun and enlightening, and may even save your life!

Jeanne Homer, M.S.
Genetic Counselor

Introduction

Ever since Alex Haley's book *Roots* was published in the 1970s, genealogy—the process of tracing your family roots—has become an intriguing hobby for many Americans. Millions of people have spent large amounts of time and money tracing their family histories to learn more about specific ancestors. This isn't surprising, given the fascination for investigating one's bloodlines. We've all thought about the possibility of finding a famous individual in our family tree. Maybe a famous politician or scientist or even a king!

But besides helping you learn whether your distant ancestor was George Washington or King Louis IX, genealogy also plays a critical role in helping you uncover your family medical history. Nearly every detail of your physical make-up and the way your body chemistry operates is determined by your genes—which have been passed down to you from the dawn of human history.

The words genealogy and genetics spring from the same linguistic root, seen in the Latin words *genus* (meaning "birth" or "descent") and *gens* (meaning "clan" or "race"). The genealogist and geneticist both set out to accomplish a similar task: finding patterns in our family relationships. Both also help us understand how we've developed into the person we are today, as well as who we will be tomorrow.

IT'S IN THE GENES

Whether we want to be or not, we're all byproducts of our biological parents—not to mention our grandparents, great-grandparents, and even more distant relatives. That's why we all frequently find ourselves thinking, "It must be in the genes." Whether it's your newborn's blue eyes that resemble her dad's, your mother's outgoing personality that reminds you of your grandfather's, or the high metabolism you inherited from your mother that allows you to eat twice as much as your friend, there's no question that we can draw many similarities between ourselves and our relatives. And if you talk to enough relatives, you'll usually discover a number of other physical characteristics and personality traits that clearly could be labeled genetic.

But aside from these most obvious hereditary traits, a closer look at your family history can reveal critical information about your present and future health. It has been proven that many of the illnesses and conditions that beset us can be predicted, diagnosed, and even prevented by studying our own family trees. As a result, increasing numbers of physicians and other health professionals recommend the need for developing thorough family health histories by tracing lineage back three or four generations.

You can't pick your genes, but knowing your family medical history can often alert you early enough to prevent a disease or minimize its effect. More than three thousand of the ten thousand known diseases and conditions have a strong hereditary component. For many years it has been known that heart disease, diabetes, hypertension, sickle cell anemia, and Huntington's chorea all have a genetic link. Recent research has also confirmed that genetics has an impact on Alzheimer's disease, multiple sclerosis, peptic ulcers, schizophrenia, depression, breast and colon cancer, retinoblastoma, and Duchenne muscular dystrophy. One startling research study even showed that children whose fathers are alcoholics are almost four times as likely to become alcoholics.

Some may think that when it comes to studying genetically caused diseases, ignorance is bliss. But it's important to remember that what you might learn in the process could actually result in better health for you and your family. It may also be of help to future generations. By understanding the genetic connection to diseases, couples contemplating having a baby can learn about the risk of having a child with a medical problem. Genetic testing both prior to and after conception gives expectant parents vital information regarding the health of their unborn baby.

SOLVING THE MYSTERIES OF DISEASE

There's another important reason for studying family health histories. If enough family trees become available for study, scientists could identify the genetic factors involved in the transmission of diseases like cancer and schizophrenia. Such a breakthrough could finally solve the mysteries of many illnesses and lead to effective new ways of preventing and treating them. In fact, mutations or changes in genes that bring about or increase the risk of certain diseases have already been identified, and in some cases genetic tests are now available that will tell you if you have that specific mutation.

The ultimate hope is that by understanding genes, specific treatments could be used to correct genetic illnesses in people who have inherited a flawed gene. By the end of 1996, nearly two hundred experiments testing various types of human gene therapy were under way in the United States. By the year 2005, scientists are expected to have mapped the entire sequence of the genetic code. This $10 billion Human Genome Project, which started in 1990 and was coordinated by the National Institute of Health (NIH), uses computerized and automated gene-mapping techniques to decipher the complex patterns of human genes. It will be many years before they know the functions of those eighty thousand genes, but ways to take advantage of this information are already being developed. It has been said that within a few decades people who feel ill will go to physician-geneticists who will run DNA scans to check the relevant genes, make diagnoses, and prescribe drugs for specific genetic needs.

YOUR FAMILY HEALTH TREE

By developing your own family health tree, you can often determine what your own risk is of developing a disease based on whether your ancestors had that same disease. The best way to record information about your family health history is to create a genogram—a graphical depiction of your relationship with your ancestors—which goes back at least three generations. A genogram (an example is shown in Figure 2, on p. 94) can reveal patterns of particular illnesses or conditions—for instance, diabetes or high blood pressure—occurring in your immediate family. It can also provide otherwise unobtainable clues for the diagnosis of illnesses. This information may enable you to prevent these illnesses years before they strike.

It's unfortunate that many of the worst diseases we suffer from are transmitted genetically. But the good news is that an accurate, detailed family tree is one of the best insurance policies you can have against illness—for yourself and your children. By knowing which illnesses you especially need to watch out for, you can take positive steps to prevent them or minimize their effect.

You will be amazed by how easy it is to construct a family health tree. The key to developing a detailed genogram that you can share with your physician is knowing where to look for information about your ancestors' health. Here's where genealogy comes into play. A wide array of information—ranging from easily obtainable government records to harder-to-find private documents—is available to anyone interested in researching their family medical history. This book will show you precisely how to access and interpret this vital information.

CLIMBING YOUR FAMILY TREE

As you create your genogram, you may start to notice patterns for specific diseases. If one of your family members has high blood pressure, it could be an isolated case. If several have had high blood pressure, you and your physician may want to analyze this more closely. If they all developed the disease at about the same age—or at a younger-than-expected age—this deserves special attention.

While recording data, it is important to consider the severity of the disease, the age of onset, and the lifestyle of the relative. For example, if your father was a vegetarian and marathon runner who was diagnosed with colon cancer at age 45 despite a healthy lifestyle, there's a good chance that genetics played a hand. If, however, he was a junk food fanatic whose only exercise consisted of getting up from the La-Z-Boy to go to the refrigerator, and he was diagnosed in his 70s, then genetics may not have been involved. Genetic counselors can help you understand the risks associated with specific illnesses and conditions.

Some medical conditions among relatives may seem random or unrelated. However, closer inspection may reveal a pattern that raises a family from average-risk to increased-risk categories. Consider cancer-syndrome families. A grandmother may have died at a young age in childbirth, but it is the three great-aunts who died of breast or ovarian cancer whose medical records would be essential for female family members who are assessing their own risks and treatment options. Information on male relatives is equally useful, even in "one sex" diseases. For example, genes that have been found for breast and ovarian cancers are not on the female sex chromosome; rather, they are on chromosomes that come from both parents. In other words, a woman can inherit a gene that increases her risk for ovarian or breast cancer from her father.

HOW TO USE THIS BOOK

When it comes to starting a family medical search, there is no better time than the present, especially since important older relatives are still alive and can remember details about their ancestors' lives and deaths. As you uncover information about your medical legacy, you'll also discover many inter-esting details about your family history, particularly if you've never conducted any genealogical research. Everybody has some fascinating ancestors in their past, hiding in the shadows of time—people whose genes are in your body now, shaping you physically, mentally, emotionally, and socially. Researching your family medical history will also help you learn more about your ancestry.

The information in this book is organized to take you step-by-step through the process of tracing your family medical history. First, we will begin with how to go about interviewing and researching your living family members. Then we'll look at how to access public and private records to learn all about your ancestors. Chapter 3 covers govern-ment sources and statistics. Chapter 4 provides information on religious and funeral records. Chapter 5 offers an overview of how to locate medical records, such as hospital and doctor's reports and insurance records, which often provide the most descriptive information about illnesses and medical conditions. Chapter 6 gives a detailed listing of libraries and archives that provide myriad resources for both amateur and advanced genealogists.

In chapter 7, you'll learn how to take all of your research and create a family health tree. Finally, chapter 8 discusses what a doctor or genetic counselor can do for you now that you have assembled your family medical history. The book closes with a look into the future of genetics.

You will find the glossaries and appendices to be an invalu-able resource. The *Glossary of Terms* will help you understand the various terms used throughout the book. The *Glossary of*

Genetic Diseases presents an overview of the most common genetic diseases and what you can do to help prevent the onset of a disease to which you might be susceptible. The appendices provide phone numbers and addresses of hundreds of private and public organizations to aid you as you conduct your research.

So how do you get started? What is considered a genetic illness? How do you create a genogram? What should be included? Where do you get the information? How can this information protect your family's health, now and in the future? Read on, and you will become an expert in tracing your family medical history! But before we begin, let's visit with some real people who took constructive steps after learning that they or their immediate family members had a genetic disorder.

CHAPTER I

Real People Facing Family Health Decisions

Note: The names of all individuals mentioned in this book have been changed to protect their identities.

Carolyn and Craig Johnson's expectation of having a healthy first baby was crushed when they learned shortly after Megan's birth that she had cystic fibrosis (CF)—one of the most common fatal genetic diseases in the United States. (Cystic fibrosis occurs in approximately one out of every fifteen hundred births and the gene is carried by an estimated one out of every twenty Caucasians.)

For the past three years, the Johnsons have done all they could to help Megan live comfortably and happily despite her disease, but last year they decided another baby—one without cystic fibrosis—would not only make their family feel more complete but would also help alleviate some of the pressure the Johnsons constantly felt from caring for an ill child.

Carolyn and Craig learned from a genetic counselor that since they were both carriers of the recessive CF gene, they had a one in four chance of having another baby with CF. Their desire to have another baby outweighed this risk, and in a short while Carolyn was pregnant for the second time. The genetic counselor advised them to take the prenatal screening test for CF, which has been available for a little over a decade. The Johnsons rejoiced when they learned from the test that this second baby was free of disease.

When Jose Fuentes' mother had a stroke at the age of 65, he realized quickly that he knew very little about his ancestors' health patterns. His grandparents had all died before he turned five, and his remaining relatives lived scattered throughout the United States and Mexico.

This need to learn more about his forebears led him to organize a family reunion in his hometown of San Diego, where 50 of his cousins, aunts, and uncles congregated to share information about their relatives. During this weekend reunion, Jose learned that heart disease was very prevalent on his mother's side of the family. This news caused Jose, 37, to take a strong look at his own lifestyle. In less than one year, he changed jobs in order to work in a less stressful environment, quit smoking, and lost 20 pounds.

Susan Coughlin was a freshman in high school 19 years ago when her mother died of breast cancer. At that time, Susan and her two older sisters had no clue regarding what lay in store for them as direct descendants of a mother who had a lethal mutation of two genes, BRCA1 and BRCA2. Together these gene mutations are probably to blame for most hereditary breast and ovarian cancers.

Now they are each confronting their genetic past in their own personal ways. Susan's sister Joanie was diagnosed with breast cancer two years ago at age 43—the same age that their mother was diagnosed with breast cancer. This happened just one year after their maternal aunt died of ovarian cancer. Susan's other sister Cathy reacted to all of this by making lifestyle changes that she hoped would lower her chances of getting breast and ovarian cancer. She lost 20 pounds, stopped drinking, and now exercises each day for 30 minutes. Susan, however, has taken a more drastic step. After paying $3,000 for the genetic test for breast cancer, she learned she had inherited her mother's flawed gene. She then decided to have both breasts removed even though she did not have breast cancer.

Sue McCarthy was only 21 and in college when she heard the shocking news from her father that her mother was diagnosed with Huntington's disease at age 55. As far as Sue knew, nobody in her family had ever suffered from this disease. However, after tracing her family medical history, she realized that both her maternal grandmother and aunt may actually have ended up contracting Huntington's disease if they hadn't died earlier in a car accident when Sue was only two. (The age of onset for Huntington's disease is usually between 35 and 45, though in rare instances it can occur earlier or later.)

For months Sue struggled with the fact that she may have inherited a genetic time bomb. Since she qualified for genetic testing of Huntington's disease, Sue decided that being tested was the only way she could go on with her life, knowing that she was either free from the disease or might soon start showing symptoms. Sue was ecstatic when the test results revealed that there was no abnormality in the gene IT-15 on chromosome 4, which is responsible for Huntington's disease. Now she is focusing on helping her mother and father.

Scott Finley was healthy when he visited a genetic cardiologist at age 45 to determine his risk for heart disease. Scott's concern was that his father had died of a heart attack at 53 and two other male relatives had also suffered from heart disease before age 60. Although all his vital readings on blood pressure and cholesterol were normal, when tested for the APOE (gene mutation for heart disease), Scott was found to have two copies of APOE, which not only gives him a 25% chance of developing heart disease, but also increases significantly his risk for Alzheimer's disease.

After getting the results, Scott suggested to his two brothers that they take the test. One made an appointment, but the other preferred not knowing what his chances were for developing either disease.

John Fletcher's brother Phil was a month shy of turning 42 when a malignant tumor was found in his colon. John, who was only 39 at the time, had never given a whole lot of thought to his family medical history. Although he had never smoked, John was a good 20 pounds overweight and seldom exercised. After hearing the news about his brother, he became more curious about the high incidence of cancer in his family, particularly since his mother had died from ovarian cancer at the age of 62. As he started interviewing relatives about other family members, he learned that his maternal grandfather had died at the age of 32 from a tumor in the colon that was situated exactly where Phil's tumor was located. Thinking that he had inherited some of these same genes from his mother and grandfather, he made an appointment for a complete physical. Thankfully, he was given a clean bill of health. He now gets colon exams on a regular basis.

These poignant stories illustrate exactly how genetics influence everyone's health. They also reveal how the knowledge of your family medical history is essential for safeguarding your own health and that of your immediate family, as well as future generations to come. Whether it involves learning more about disease patterns in your family, deciding to have a genetic test to determine your own or your child's risk of developing a disease, or taking more extreme measures by having elective prophylactic (preventive) surgery to avoid future problems, understanding more about your family medical history is your first step toward living a healthier life. In today's world, where new information becomes available almost weekly about disease and genetics, being forewarned means being forearmed.

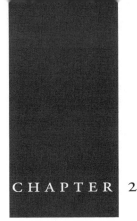

CHAPTER 2

Your Family: Your Best Resource

Americans are hardly strangers to unearthing family history. Many people have dabbled in genealogy and tens of millions have compiled some form of a family tree. Still, even with all this interest in family roots, few people know even the barest details of their relatives' medical histories. They may remember that Uncle Joe died of some form of heart disease before age 50, but they might not recall specifically what the diagnosis was.

Where does one get accurate information about family illnesses? Not from old tombstones or family Bibles in Germany. Those sources are helpful if you're compiling a family tree that spans many centuries. However, in tracing your family medical history, you need not go back seven generations. It is true that the further back you can trace, the more helpful it can be; but what's more important is obtaining accurate, relevant medical information that will help you uncover specific family predispositions to illness. This kind of health information can be found if you focus on the past three or four generations.

One of the problems for most people is that they don't know where to start to obtain family medical histories. Family, in this context, means relatives related by blood, rather than by marriage or adoption. For example, if two uncles had spouses who died from breast cancer, it might superficially appear as though their family was at risk. However, for blood relatives of the uncles, there would be no increase in the likelihood of contracting breast cancer.

Surprisingly, the first place to begin your search for your family medical history is also probably your easiest resource: your living relatives, starting with your mother and father. After interviewing your most immediate family members, you then need to branch out and talk to less directly related relatives, even third and fourth cousins. Remember, the best family medical histories have more width than depth.

It's a good idea to give the person enough time to prepare for the interview. Ask them a week in advance to start gathering photos, letters, documents, or other items that will help them share memories with you. A long-lost photograph often serves as a trigger for memories long-forgotten.

While interviewing your parents and other relatives, you may want to use a tape recorder so you can transcribe the conversation later. Small, portable tape recorders are inexpensive, and their built-in microphones are unobtrusive. Check your equipment to make sure you have enough tape, batteries, and other accessories for the interview. By taping the conversation, you will be able to concentrate on what the person is saying rather than trying to write down every word that comes up. Plus, the tape will become a valuable heirloom for you to share with other family members and future generations. You might even consider videotaping the interview. If you use a tripod, you won't have to worry about the mechanics of videotaping the interview and you will be able to concentrate on the discussion.

A questionnaire (shown in Figure 1, on p. 28) can also help you in asking the right questions. Some people are a little uncomfortable talking about personal health issues, so the questionnaire may be a useful tool in helping to break the ice. When writing up your questions, try to order them in such a way that one question leads naturally into the next. For instance, if you want to know about one relative in particular, keep all your questions about this person— when he was born, how he died, etc.—together so you are not jumping back and forth from one person or subject to another. You should also avoid questions that elicit a simple yes or no response. The whole idea is to learn as much as possible from these personal interviews.

Don't be surprised if you need to go back later to a family member to ask more specific questions. Often the original questions are too broad and may require more details. For example, during the first discussion your mother might tell you that Aunt Birdie died from breast cancer. But after thinking about it for a while, you might realize that you should've asked if your aunt had also suffered from angina.

FIGURE I

QUESTIONNAIRE FOR OBTAINING FAMILY HEALTH INFORMATION

1. What was the date of death for my relatives—going back four generations? (If you can't obtain exact dates, ask about the approximate years.)

2. What was their age at death?

3. Where were they born, and where did they later reside?

4. What was their cause of death?

5. What was the age of onset of a specific illness?

6. Did these relatives have any other known diseases? If so, when was the onset of these illnesses?

7. Did any of my relatives smoke? Did any abuse alcohol or prescription/illicit drugs?

8. Were there any known miscarriages or stillbirths?

9. Did any of my relatives have a history of mental illness or were they institutionalized?

10. What were the general physical characteristics of my relatives, particularly related to height, weight, and skin color? What was their race and religion?

A FAMILY TREE PARTY

If you have an extremely close family, you may want to consider having a family tree party or reunion. You may find that some of your relatives have already conducted some genealogical studies and have found some useful family medical information during the process. By gathering everyone together at one time, it's not only fast and effective, but it's also a lot of fun! It's a common tendency to think your relatives are too busy to want to attend a family reunion; but you'll be surprised by the enthusiastic response you'll receive if you make the effort to put a reunion together.

As you plan for this reunion, include uncles, aunts, cousins, second cousins, parents, grandparents, great-aunts, and great-uncles—as many relatives as you can reasonably trace and invite. If possible, explain the purpose of the gathering in the invitation, so people can think about the health information needed beforehand.

You may be able to name your immediate family forebears, for at least a couple of generations, but most people know surprisingly little about their grandparents' families and even less about their great-grandparents. Older relatives will help fill in some of this information, while your cousins can help you expand your genogram sideways.

It's important to remember that unless many of your family members are doctors or geneticists, the information they provide may be inaccurate and the terminology may be incorrect. You still should write down the information as stated, but then verify it later with additional research. Older relatives can become confused about specific cases.

Aunt Cecilia may consider herself an expert on knowing all about the family tree, when in fact she could have everything mixed up. She may tell you, for example, that your great-grandfather had suffered from a stroke, when it really was your great-grandmother.

The embarrassment and dread of many illnesses and conditions in the past—such as cancer, Alzheimer's disease and suicide—have caused many older individuals to talk about these conditions in hushed tones, if they are even mentioned at all. Many people might say that a relative died "after a long illness" instead of stating the specific cause of the death. Some family members do not want it to be known that one family member had five miscarriages or that a cousin who died "after a long illness" actually died of AIDS. Sensitivity and discretion must be applied in these circumstances.

On some occasions, the diagnosis the doctor had initially given the family turns out to be wrong, even though clarification was never given to relatives. For example, adverse reactions to drugs sometimes produce symptoms that mimic those of a chronic disorder, such as Alzheimer's disease. Check with as many relatives as you can about the health histories of deceased loved ones. Sometimes these stories may vary.

INTERVIEWING TIPS

Since you will be asking family members personal questions, it's important to make them feel as comfortable as possible. You must make it clear why sensitive questions are being posed. Explain thoroughly why this project is crucial for you, your relative, and future generations in your family.

You should also try to make the discussion more enjoyable by asking for anecdotes and personality descriptions. Relatives love sharing these stories with family members. You may even learn a thing or two about your family during this process. Good listening skills are essential when interviewing relatives. Never interrupt and don't assume someone has finished just because they pause for a moment. Wait for the person to tell you he is finished or wait for a substantial pause before you start your next question. Even if the relative starts wandering and talks about things you haven't asked him about, let him keep talking. He may end up revealing some interesting facts about your family history, whether it's health-related or not.

The following questions should prove useful in starting your discussion:

- Can you think of any traits running in our family that seem unusual?
- Were any of our relatives extremely tall or of short stature? Were any obese or extremely thin?
- Were there any miscarriages or stillbirths? (This can provide information about possible problem pregnancies.)
- Did any family members have reconstructive surgery, i.e., for repair of cleft palate?
- Were there any learning disabilities or speech problems?
- What types of allergies, whether hay fever, reactions to food, anesthesia, or medications, did family members experience?
- Who suffered from major diseases? (See Figure 4, on p. 103 for list)

- What was the age of onset for these diseases? (Diabetes that strikes a teenager is quite different from that which appears at the age of 65.)
- Did anyone abuse alcohol or drugs?
- Which relatives smoked? How much and for how long?
- Did anyone suffer from recurring headaches, frequent colds, or even limps?
- Did any relative commit suicide or suffer from depression?
- Did any of your relatives marry cousins?

YOUR GRANDMA'S ATTIC: A TREASURE TROVE OF INFORMATION

If your relatives do not provide you with enough information through interviews, your other option is to search through any family heirlooms or records that may have been stored away. If possible, try to gain access to their attics or basements, where you may uncover long-forgotten, but often valuable, photographs and mementos. A photograph can provide important information about physical characteristics, such as the weight and height of your relatives.

Each of your relatives has created his or her own paper trail: a birth and baptismal certificate, school records, photographs, marriage certificates, military records, insurance papers, deeds and wills, and employment records. When this information is analyzed for a number of your relatives, you will gain a better understanding of your entire family. Here are some things you should look for:

Family Bibles—Since early American tradition stipulated that the Bible hold vital family information and records, family Bibles are an excellent source for information on marriages, births, and deaths. The same holds true for many other sacred texts, representing religions around the world. Many records are handwritten right inside the front cover or on the first one or two pages. When studying this information, always compare the publication date of the Bible with the date of the entry or date of birth of the person who recorded the information. This way you'll be able to tell if the material was entered after the fact, or if it is firsthand information. The handwriting of the entries can also provide you with valuable clues: if it is uniform throughout, then the chances are good that one person entered the information in one sitting, from memory or secondhand and third-hand information, long after the actual births and deaths of the parties involved.

Personal Diaries—Although diaries might not provide a lot of specific health-related information about your relatives, they are a rich biographical resource.

Family Records—A variety of legal documents can provide a great deal of insight into your roots. Look specifically for birth and death certificates, insurance papers, wills, church records, health papers, military papers, documented family histories, yearbooks, and passports.

Miscellaneous Items—Once you start looking, you will be amazed at some of the relics you'll uncover. Art work or furniture with inscriptions and dates, scrapbooks, baby books, old letters, newspaper clippings, trophies, and invitations all provide an intriguing glimpse into your family's past.

PROBING FOR MORE DETAILS

Once you've found out which relatives had experienced specific diseases, you need to probe a little deeper for additional details. For example, if you learn that a family member has diabetes, it is important to learn at what age it was diagnosed, how it was treated, and if there are any other family members with diabetes. If this individual was the only member of the family with diabetes, it was probably an isolated case. If several relatives had diabetes, it takes on greater importance.

You should always ask how old the relative was when he got sick. As a rule, the earlier the age of onset, the more likely that the condition was due to inherited genes. For instance, if your mother had an illness like breast cancer, heart disease, or hypertension before menopause, your risk will be higher than if she had developed the disorder after menopause began.

As you interview your relatives, you should inquire about the ethnicity of certain family members. Some ethnic groups are likelier than others to develop specific diseases. For instance, many Ashkenazi Jews have suffered from genetic disorders that can be traced back through their ancestry. It's also important to inquire about possible environmental factors that may have affected them. The cause of heart disease is estimated to be about 60% environmental—lack of exercise, cigarette smoking, too much fat in the diet, emotional stress, etc. So if you learn that a relative suffered from heart disease at the age of 55, it's important to check on these environmental factors in case they were to blame.

Through your research you may find certain conditions that on the surface don't appear to be possible genetic disorders. Your Uncle Jim had numerous broken bones, supposedly caused by accidents. At least that's what your mother told you. But if you consult with a genetic counselor or doctor, you will learn that a tendency to break bones frequently can be an indication of certain groups of genetically inherited bone disorders.

Occasionally, there may be hidden information in what appears to be ordinary material. For instance, your mother may tell you she had an uncle who was deaf but neglect to tell you that his deafness was caused by rubella (German measles). This missing information is critical because rubella does not have any genetic links.

Always ask about the reason for blindness (which is 50% genetic), deafness, surgery, muscle weakness, and mental retardation (which may be from an accident, infection, or high fever rather than a chromosomal or genetic cause).

As you research specific individuals, dig for as much information as possible. If a grandmother died of a stroke, was it caused by a blood clot or by bleeding in the brain? Did she also have high blood pressure? What was her diet like? If she died of cancer, what type was it?

After you have conducted all of these interviews, you'll be surprised at the amount of data that emerges. Those individuals with close relationships to many relatives, including elderly relatives who are still alive, will probably end up with almost enough information to make their genograms complete. Others who only come up with the basics—known medical conditions, symptoms, and signs—

may still have to do a little more digging. Chapters 3–6 will assist you in that area. Regardless, by interviewing your living relatives, you are now one step closer to making a significant difference in your family's health and well-being.

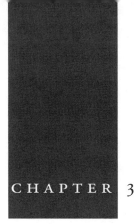

CHAPTER 3

Government Sources

After gathering as much information as possible from your living relatives, you are ready to start investigating the medical history of remaining family members, many of whom may go back several generations. A variety of resources are available to help you in your search. Many of the records you will study may not contain specific health information about your relatives, but they will be necessary in locating those ancestors who play a genetic role in shaping your life. For instance, a marriage license will not tell you how healthy your great-great-aunt was, but it will shed some light on who this individual was and how she is related to you.

Both the federal and state governments maintain a number of records that will assist you in tracing your family medical history. As you start your research, you'll be surprised how much you can learn about yourself and your family from these official documents. Not only will you be able to start piecing together family health information, you'll also uncover some intriguing facts about your ancestors. You may even end up enjoying genealogy so much that it will become one of your favorite hobbies!

DEATH CERTIFICATES

Death certificates—which are original documents that are created at the time of someone's death—are one of your most valuable resources for tracing family medical histories. Most death certificates are available from state government offices, called vital statistics offices, which are usually part of each state's Department of Health and Social Services. The names of these offices vary from state to state, but for the most part, a Bureau of Vital Statistics located in the capital city will have these records. Death certificates are kept in the state where the deceased passed away, not where they were buried.

A death certificate can be a useful tool because it might include the primary and secondary causes of death (for example, heart failure as the primary cause and carcinoma of the lung as the secondary cause), the date of the onset of the illness, and surgeries that were performed as part of the treatment. Death certificates can also contain the names of the deceased's parents, which you will need if you are going to search back another generation. Other information may include the name of the doctor, place of death, usual residence, name of hospital, name of mortician, name and location of cemetery, occupation, marital status, and name of spouse. Most death certificates are filled out by an attending physician, which means the information is usually accurate and valuable to other physicians in diagnosing possible conditions in your family.

In order to compile an accurate family health tree, you should obtain death certificates for all parents, grandparents, and their siblings. Your grandmother may have died from a non-genetic disease or an accident, even though all of her sisters suffered from diabetes and breast cancer.

American death certificates have not been standardized. Therefore, you will find that some death certificates are very sparse while others are full of details. One death certificate may show that your ancestor Robert Green died on 25 August 1911 at Kankakee (Kankakee County, Illinois) of a stroke. His doctor was B.A. Critten of the same town. Green was a white male, age 46, an American citizen, born in America, and a resident of Kankakee. The record indicated no next of kin, survivors, or parents' names.

The next record, however, which lists the 1927 death of your relative Laurel O'Connor gives a lot more information. She was a white female, age 68 years, 10 months, and 13 days, born on 18 June 1859 in New York City, New York, who had lived for 30 years in Boston prior to moving to New York City. She was the widow of Kenneth Wells and her parents' names were Scott and Catherine Riley. She died at 10 p.m. of congestive heart failure, complicated by pneumonia, which was documented by her physician, Thomas Lindley, M.D. The mortuary was O'Farrell-Green Company on Canal Street, New York City, and burial was at Saint Mary's Cemetery on May 6. This more detailed record would allow you to search further by contacting the funeral home or cemetery.

Death certificates can be very useful, but you should remember that they are still secondhand sources of birth information. You must be aware of the possibility that birthdate, birthplace, or parents' names and birthplaces may be incorrect. Therefore, it's best if you can verify this information from another source. There will be misdiagnoses on both current and past death certificates due to a variety of reasons. Many medical conditions were not medically understood in the past. Today, misleading information can result from incompetence and an unfortunate trend of not performing enough autopsies. Sometimes there will even be lies brought on by embarrassment. For instance, pneumonia might be listed instead of AIDS, and suicide may go unidentified due to the family's request, religious beliefs, or life-insurance claims.

Sometimes, if you go back several generations and find a death certificate, there may be incomplete information because the relative died at home and there were no medical records. Some death certificates might cite a tumor, but the location is not given. If this was your relative, you would want to do some more investigative work, especially if she died under the age of 50.

To send for copies of death certificates, refer to Appendix B, on page 177. The cost of copies and years available vary from state to state. Costs for certified copies range from about $5 to as much as $30; therefore, obtaining one for all of the relatives you are tracking can be expensive. You should check first to see if any copies of death certificates exist among family members. This will save you money and eliminate obtaining duplicate copies. You should also inquire about getting a copy of a death certificate instead of a certified copy, which costs more. You are just interested in reading the information from the record, not using it for any legal purposes.

The dates that are available for death certificates will also vary from state to state. Some states, like Delaware, have death records that date from as early as 1861, but the majority of state records begin in the early 1900s.

Death records are sometimes available at county courthouses or city halls. Some cities initiated birth and death registration before their states did and therefore maintain their own records. In some cities, births and deaths that occur within city limits are registered with the city rather than the county. Some of this country's older cities have death records dating back as far as 1803 (New Orleans) or 1875 (Baltimore). Since copies of death certificates at the local level are often less expensive than at the state level, you should try to find records there first if you know the city or county where the person died.

If one of your relatives was a U.S. citizen and died in a foreign country, the death would normally have been reported to the nearest U.S. consular office. The consul in that foreign country would have prepared an official "Report of the Death of an American Citizen Abroad" and a copy of the report of death would have been permanently filed with the U.S. Department of State. To obtain a copy of a report, write to Passport Services, Correspondence Branch, U.S. Department of State, Washington, DC 20523.

If your ancestor was a member of the armed forces of the United States at the time of his death, the records will be in another location. For members of the Army, Navy, or Air Force, write to the Secretary of Defense, Washington, DC 20301. For members of the Coast Guard, write to the Commandant, P.S., U.S. Coast Guard, Washington, DC 20226.

When a death occurs on the high seas, whether in an aircraft or on a vessel, the determination of where the record is filed is decided by the direction in which the aircraft or vessel was heading at the time of the event. If it was outbound or docked or landed at a foreign port, requests for copies of the records should be made to the U.S. Department of State, Washington, DC 20520. If it was inbound and the first port of entry was the United States, you should write to the registration authority in the city where the vessel or aircraft docked or landed in the United States.

Most foreign countries record births and deaths and most will provide certificates of birth and death occurring within their boundaries. U.S. citizens who need a copy of a foreign death record may obtain assistance by writing to the Office of Overseas Citizens Services, U.S. Department of State, Washington, DC 20520.

If you need additional information about obtaining death records, these are excellent resources that should provide help:

—*Vital Records Handbook*, by Thomas J. Kemp (Baltimore: Genealogical Publishing Company, 1989). This gives a state-by-state listing of agencies, costs for records, limitations or restrictions, and the necessary forms that may be photocopied.

—*International Vital Records Handbook* (same author and publisher, 1994) is an expanded edition, covering 67 countries and territories, including the United States.

—*Where to Write for Vital Records: Births, Deaths, Marriages and Divorces* (Hyattsville, MD: U.S. Department of Health and Human Services, Public Health Service, 1993 or later edition). Gives agency, address, and availability of records for states and territories as well as records of citizens born "on the high seas" or in foreign countries.

MORTALITY SCHEDULES (1850–85)

The federal government kept mortality schedules between the years 1850 and 1885, and they were developed for the purpose of collecting information about births, marriages, and deaths. Mortality schedules predate the registration of vital statistics at the turn of the century and can be extremely useful in compiling data about the cause of death of some of your ancestors.

These schedules list deaths for the 12 months prior to the census. For example, the mortality schedule of 1878 would record deaths from June 1, 1877 through May 31, 1878. However, there are exceptions to these dates, so you should check the schedules if any of your relatives died any time during the 1849 to 1850 time period. Typically the information contained in the schedules includes the name of the person, his or her age, sex, state of birth, month of death, profession/occupation/trade, and number of days ill. In the 1880 mortality schedule, the place where the disease was contracted, the nature of the illness, and the name of the attending physician were all added.

Interestingly, slaves were named in these schedules, but there is no surname, and the slave owner's name is not specified. If a slave owner reported a death in his own family and any deaths among his slaves at the same time, the deceased persons could be listed on consecutive lines of the schedule page.

Although you may find some interesting genealogical tidbits from mortality schedules, you may not find a lot of accurate health reporting. During the years covered in the schedules, common causes of death were consumption, pneumonia, diarrhea and related conditions, fevers of various kinds (typhoid, malaria, etc.), drowning and accidental wounds, childbirth, and various heart-related conditions. It wasn't even unusual to include causes such as "congestion of the brain" or "softening of the brain." Still, you shouldn't overlook mortality schedules as a source of information that may lead you to other more accurate records.

Many of the original mortality schedules are stored at the National Archives or in state governmental agencies. Those not claimed by the states were given to the National Society of the Daughters of the American Revolution (DAR) and were placed in its library in Washington, DC. The original schedules held by DAR are for the states of Arizona, Colorado, Georgia, Kentucky, Louisiana, Tennessee, and the District of Columbia. Most of these have been indexed by DAR and some have been transcribed.

The federal mortality schedules for Arizona, Colorado, District of Columbia, Georgia, Kentucky, Louisiana, and Tennessee have been reproduced as microfilm publication T655, Federal Mortality Census Schedules, 1850–1880, and Related Indexes in the Custody of the Daughters of the American Revolution. This microfilm publication is found at the Chicago, Denver, and Los Angeles branches of the National Archives. Other branch collections of mortality schedules on microfilm or in printed form include Iowa (1850–80), Nebraska (1860 and 1870), Kansas (1860–80) at the Kansas City branch, and Virginia (1850–80) at the Philadelphia branch.

Consult the Guide to Genealogical Research in the National Archives (Washington, DC: National Archives, 1985) for a list of mortality schedules by state available through the National Archives and its regional branches.

Most mortality schedules are also available through the Church of Jesus Christ of Latter-Day Saints (abbreviated LDS) Family History Library in Salt Lake City, Utah, and its hundreds of branches throughout the country, and will be found on microfiche. To determine the ones available, check the Family History Library Catalog at any branch library under [State]/Census or [State]/Vital Records.

Mortality schedules will help you trace and document genetic symptoms and diseases. By using this information to record death dates of family members, you can then follow up with focused searches in obituaries, mortuary records, and cemeteries.

CENSUS RECORDS

By definition, a census is a counting of people. The first federal censuses were introduced by the British government during the colonial period. While censuses date back to this period, for the purpose of obtaining information about your family's health, the ones you probably will be most concerned with are fairly recent—dating back from 1920 (the most recent available to the public at this date) to 1850. By law, these documents are kept confidential for 72 years after each census. Census records before 1900 are rather sketchy, but if you know the names of ancestors who lived in this country from 1900 to 1920, you might be able to find some interesting information.

Since the 1920, 1910, and 1900 censuses are the most valuable, you should begin your research with them. These records are available in the National Archives in Washington, DC, and in all 11 of its regional branches located in the metropolitan areas of Atlanta, Boston, Chicago, Denver, Fort Worth, Kansas City, Los Angeles, New York City, Philadelphia, San Francisco, and Seattle.

1920 CENSUS

The 1920 Federal Population Census was released in 1992 and is currently available for all the states. This census also includes the military and naval population living abroad. Even though the medical history is lacking in this census report, you will learn interesting facts, such as the names of individuals in each household, their birthdates, birth places of parents and the language of the parents. There is also additional information about each person's education, ability to read and write, and occupational data, along with other personal identifying information.

1910 CENSUS

Although the 1910 Federal Population Census also asked a number of questions that will provide vital information about your family, the questions relating to health were minimal. It asked if a person was blind in both eyes or deaf and dumb. Answers to these questions pertaining to family members may give you clues to possible genetic diseases that run in your family. But don't forget that blindness and genetic diseases could have been the result of accidents or other diseases and might not be genetic in origin.

If, however, you discover a number of your ancestors were listed as blind after they reached middle age, the cause could have been glaucoma, which has been linked genetically. Likewise, if a number of ancestors had been listed as being deaf, modern records may back up the fact that these distant relatives suffered from a genetic hearing condition.

1900 CENSUS

The 1900 Census does not contain much information useful for a family health tree other than how many children your female ancestor gave birth to and how many were living in 1900. It may, however, give you some indication of female-related problems if you discover your ancestor gave birth to 10 children but only one or two survived. Even though that isn't sufficient proof that the woman experienced reproduction problems—remember, there were many childhood diseases at that time—it may be worth investigating a little further to rule out female, genetically linked conditions.

1890 CENSUS

Unfortunately, this census was almost completely destroyed in a fire in 1921 and only portions of it exist. This was a major loss, since this census asked about chronic or acute diseases and whether an individual was crippled, maimed, or deformed (with name of defect). The surviving information has been indexed and both the census and the index were microfilmed, and they are available at all branches of the National Archives. You might be able to find some information on your relatives from this resource.

1880 CENSUS

The 1880 Census allows you to begin tracing some of your family medical history. It asked about illness or disability on the day of the census and is the first census to state everyone's relationship to the head of the household. It also asked whether persons were deaf, dumb, blind, or insane.

1870 CENSUS

The 1870 Census asked whether a person was deaf, dumb, blind, or insane and whether a person was a survivor of the Civil War, which can lead you to the military and pension records that may contain family medical information.

MILITARY RECORDS

The military records of some of your ancestors may provide information about the diseases from which they suffered. To obtain copies of records of veterans who served before World War I, use NATF Form 80, available from the National Archives, to request a search of the records. Complete the form and mail to: Military Service Branch (NNMS), National Archives and Records Service, 8th and Pennsylvania Avenue, N.W., Washington, DC 20408.

Service and pension records for those who served during World War I can be obtained by writing to: The National Archives, Atlanta Branch, 1557 St. Joseph Avenue, East Point,

GA 30344. Service and pension records for those who served after World War I are not available for public viewing, though some information can be obtained under certain conditions. Most of the federal records in this category are housed at the National Personnel Records Center, 9700 Page Boulevard, St. Louis, MO 63123. Living veterans can request their records or give written consent to others.

The following publications provide more specific information on conducting historical military research:

—*U.S. Military Records* (Family History Library, 1993). Describes the various types of military records, lists the resources available to researchers at the library in Salt Lake City or through its branch libraries.

—*U.S. Military Records: A Guide to Federal and State Sources, Colonial America to the Present* by James C. Neagles. Describes the various types of military records and continues with post-service records and the records of the National Archives, its regional branches, and its repositories.

IMMIGRATION

Written records of immigrants date back about five hundred years, and the majority of them cover only about two hundred to two hundred fifty years. But, obviously, for tracing your family medical history, this is more than adequate, since you don't have to go back more than several generations. Don't expect to find any health information in immigration records, but they will help you determine where specific ancestors may have come from. Then you can track down more health-related data from those countries.

If specific ancestors arrived in the United States by ship after 1820, there might be a record of their arrival in The National Archives in Washington, DC. A staff member of the Archives will search through the records for you if you know the name of your ancestor, the year and month of their arrival, and the name of the ship they took. If you know only the name of the ancestor, you can go to the main branch of The National Archives or any regional branch and begin the search yourself. You should ask for Form 81 to apply for a copy of the ship's manifest. (See Appendix A, on p. 175, for addresses and locations of the National Archives and its regional branches.)

For those ancestors who emigrated into eastern U.S. seaports—the Port of New York and other eastern seaboard ports since 1891—you should contact: The United States Department of Justice, Immigration and Naturalization Service, Records and Verification Center, 1446-21 Edwin Miller Boulevard, Martinsburg, WV 25401.

If your ancestor became a citizen after 1906, you will probably find a record of her at the Immigration and Naturalization Service (INS) Office. You should contact them and make a request under the Freedom of Information Act/ Privacy Act. Ask for Form G-639. Write to: Immigration and Naturalization Service, FOIA/PA Office, Washington, DC, 20536.

Specific publications containing records of immigration can also be helpful in conducting your search. Some of the best are:

—*Passenger and Immigration Lists Index (PILI): A Guide to Published Arrival Records of About 500,000 Passengers Who*

Came to the United States and Canada in the Seventeenth, Eighteenth and Nineteenth Centuries by P. William Filby (Detroit: Gale Research, 1981). This multivolume bibliography and index includes more than 2 million names from published passenger lists and naturalization records. Each entry gives age, place, year of arrival, and names of family members.

—*Passenger and Immigration Lists Bibliography, 1538–1900* by P. William Filby is the companion book to the above-mentioned resource. This bibliography helps the researcher by indexing ethnic groups, destinations, and arrival ports and states.

—*Immigrant and Passenger Arrivals: A Select Catalog of National Archives Microfilm Publications* (Washington, DC: National Archives, 2nd edition, 1991). Some of the lists in this record include crew members on the vessels, which might be of interest when trying to find out who emigrated with specific ancestors.

PASSPORT RECORDS

Early passport records were used domestically, allowing U.S. citizens to travel between states and territories. These documents contain the individual's name, date of birth, where he lives, and a photograph (after the advent of photography). Once again, these records won't include health information on your ancestors, but they will help you learn where they lived.

In recent years, U.S. passport records from the first half of the century have been moved to different locations. In late 1993, the National Archives in Washington, DC, received passports issued between 1789 and 1905, and the Washington National Records Center in Suitland, Maryland, received those issued between 1906 and 1925. Because of the relocation of these records, you should write or call in advance to determine the location of the records you need to study.

In the early 20th century, U.S. consulates abroad started registering the names, dates of birth, and birthplaces of all U.S. citizens living in foreign countries. Available through the National Archives, these records could be crucial in your research if one of your ancestors spent a few years outside of the U.S.

SOCIAL SECURITY ADMINISTRATION RECORDS

The United States Social Security Death Index (about 1935 forward) is available on CD-ROM in the Family History Centers (see p. 84) and other research libraries. By entering the name of the deceased relative, you can learn birth and death dates, place where the Social Security card was issued, Social Security number, and residence of the person at the time of death. Although extensive, this index is not complete. Obtaining the same type of information from the Social Security Administration takes more time, but records are more complete. The application for a Social Security number contains such information as full name, birth date and place, and sometimes parents' names, spouse's name, and employment information. The death date may be included if the number was issued in order to process survivor benefits. Claims filed may also contain death and survivor information. Since the form was usually completed by the applicant, parent, or spouse, it can be a reliable source for general genealogical research.

Local branch offices of the Social Security Administration have access to these records, which were recently computerized. Although some local offices may agree to handle requests for this information by mail, others require that you appear in person.

The documentation necessary for them to release information is your ID, the ancestor's Social Security number and whatever it takes to prove your relationship to that person, such as a series of birth certificates showing your descent from that ancestor.

MARRIAGE RECORDS

Marriage records will not give you specific health information about your ancestors, but they are helpful with the general tracing of roots. They can give you facts about where an ancestor resided at a particular date. Some marriage records were filed in counties that required more detailed information, such as names of parents and family members, where the bride and groom resided prior to marriage, and where their parents were born.

Marriage documents are vital records usually found in county courthouses, with copies often in the state library, archives, or historical society. In some states, the records are also being centralized in the state vital statistics or vital records office, but the county courthouse is where the license is issued and the record is generated. The particular office in the county courthouse where the records are kept varies from county clerk to probate clerk or circuit court clerk. Two resources—Kemp's *Vital Records Handbook* and the U.S. Department of Health and Human Services' *Where to Write for Vital Records: Births, Deaths, Marriages and Divorces* (both mentioned previously on p. 42)—will assist you in locating the appropriate offices.

ADOPTION RECORDS

Not only do adopted individuals need to know about their biological roots, but their children and grandchildren want, and need, to know, too. It can be difficult for adoptees and their descendants to compile a comprehensive family health tree, but they should at least be able to obtain information about specific hereditary diseases and genetic traits their biological parents may have passed on to them.

Adoptees who want to learn more about their family medical history should start with their adoptive parents. They will have some knowledge of the people, places, and dates involved. States also have a central adoption unit where files are kept on all surrenders and adoptions initiated or concluded there. The records are slightly different from year to year and state to state, but they will probably include the following:

- original certificate of birth
- amended certificate of birth
- relinquishment, consent, and surrender papers
- petition to adopt
- case or home study information
- final adoption decree

Each state's centralized vital records office in the capital city will probably house these records. However, county and city bureaus still exist and often have older or duplicate records.

Unfortunately, the documents and records that an adoptee needs most to learn about his or her family medical history are the very ones that are most difficult to obtain. For instance, the original birth certificate, which is issued shortly after delivery and prior to adoption being finalized, often contains valuable information on the birth family. It may include the birth mother's maiden name, the birth father's name, their occupations, previous births to this mother, and the name of the doctor or other person attending the birth.

When an adoption is finalized, the original birth certificate is closed or "sealed" and an amended certificate is issued in its place. State laws vary on the availability of the original certificate. The original birth record may be held by city, county, or state vital records offices as well as the agency, the state department concerned, and the court. Finding this document can be one of the most challenging tasks for an adoptee searching for more family health information. Some individuals have even hired professionals to assist them.

Surrender, relinquishment, or consent to adopt documents, or copies of them, can be found in the court, agency, or state department files. The lawyer for the petitioners will usually have copies of these documents in their files. These documents will give the birth parents' names, possibly the child's birth name, the agency involved, and usually an address of the birth parent.

Fortunately, a system has been established by the International Soundex Reunion Register (ISRR), a reunion registry for adoptees, so that birth parents can warn their adopted children anonymously about diseases or conditions that could affect the child and his or her children. This medical alert and genetic outreach program has provided vital health information to thousands of adopted individuals. In the past, a girl who becomes pregnant at age 15 probably doesn't know anything about her own medical history, let alone her family's. However, by the time she is 25 or 35, she may have acquired information that should be passed on to her adopted child.

An example of how this information can help adopted children is the case of Sharon Grambs, who was adopted at birth, and knew that her birth mother had died young of a long illness. When Sharon was 29, she felt the need to research her own genetic health history. After a very lengthy process through the court system, she learned that her mother had died of ovarian cancer when she was only 42. She also learned that she had two older biological sisters: one who had suffered from uterine cancer and another who is currently experiencing a precancerous condition in her cervix. This new information led Sharon to make drastic changes to her lifestyle in terms of diet and drinking, and after her doctor's urging, she gets annual mammograms.

The following organization should provide additional information for adoptees searching for family medical information: Adoptees Liberty Movement Association (ALMA), Post Office Box 154, Washington Bridge Station, New York, New York 10033.

When you start contacting governmental agencies, it may become a little overwhelming at first. Government is a bureaucracy, which means matters are not always handled most expeditiously. Keep good notes of whom you've spoken to on the phone and, if possible, make copies of all requests for information you have mailed to different sources. This will help you keep track of the flow of information, as well as indicate which people you need to follow up with in case there appears to be a delay. And whatever you do, don't expect to obtain all this information overnight. This will become a gradual learning experience, and hopefully an interesting one too, as you uncover your family heritage.

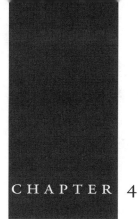

CHAPTER 4

Religious and Funeral Records

Religious records for genealogical purposes take on all forms. Some come directly from your ancestor's place of worship or the national institution associated with it. Some come from other denominations that have focused more extensively on genealogical research. One of the most noted religious institutions for this has been the Church of Jesus Christ of Latter-Day Saints, whose Genealogical Society of Utah is an unparalleled resource with a computerized index of 60 million immigrants in its Family History Library (see chapter 6, on p. 81). When searching for records, consider all religious institutions as libraries. They maintain records for births, christenings, confirmations, bar mitzvahs, bat mitzvahs, marriages, and deaths.

FAMILY RELIGIOUS RECORDS

Sometimes locating useful information about your ancestors' past is as simple as finding a family Bible or other sacred text. Many records are handwritten right into the book. You should also contact officials at cemeteries, churches, temples, or any other places your ancestor may have worshipped and ask if they have any records of your family name or names. If you learn the name of the town where your ancestor is buried (from the death certificate or other sources), then contact houses of worship and cemeteries in that town.

CEMETERY AND
FUNERAL RECORDS

Cemetery records (often called sexton's records) usually contain information about the cause of death. You should check the sexton's office in the cemetery where your ancestor was buried to see what information is available. Even some tombstones or markers identify the cause of death. If you are unable to travel to the cemetery, you can always ask somebody at the cemetery to take a picture of the tombstone and have it mailed to you.

Your more challenging task will be to learn the name of the cemetery where certain ancestors are buried. In this situation, you have several options. First, newspaper obituaries, death certificates, family Bibles and other records, family members, county and local histories, church registers, club or lodge records, and funeral home files may supply the name of the cemetery. If not, you may find transcribed cemetery records arranged by counties and states. Many are indexed by organizations such as the Family History Library, which makes them very easy to research. Some repositories have card indexes to cemeteries.

If you at least know the county in which the person resided at the time of death, you can begin by focusing on the cemeteries in that county. If no transcriptions exist for that county, you can obtain a map that shows the known cemeteries. Once again, you can either visit the cemeteries or call and ask them about your deceased ancestors. Some cemeteries have associations that keep the records or take care of the grounds. They also have maps that identify the burials in each plot. These plot maps can even indicate where and when a person was buried even if there is no tombstone to mark the spot.

Most people don't find tombstones for all of their ancestors. Purchasing gravestones was considered very expensive, especially at the turn of the century. Therefore, many family groups would pool their money to remember relatives by erecting markers.

As you investigate cemeteries as a possible resource, do not pin all your hopes on obtaining information from tombstones. Some do not even give complete birth and death dates, and most do not give the cause of death. Your best bet would be to check with cemetery officials to see what information they have on file.

OBITUARIES

Obituaries today do not usually identify the disease or illness that contributed to the cause of death, but older newspapers' obituaries usually do. Because many of these earlier obituaries contain so much detailed information, it makes sense for you to search for as many obituaries of family members as possible.

Obituaries are also a great source for learning the names and places of residence of family members, parents' names, dates of birth and death, religious affiliation, and locations of the cemetery and funeral home. In more modern obituaries, an important clue is the charity that the family requests donations for, such as the American Heart Association and the American Cancer Society. While not reliable as the cause of death, these notations may be an indication that your ancestor died or suffered from heart disease or cancer, for example.

The obituaries of most newspapers can be found on microfilm. The original issues of some newspapers may be available at county courthouses, public and university libraries, historical societies, state archives, or libraries.

The best way to determine where to find the newspapers that still exist for your research area is to consult union catalogs. Such union lists identify which libraries or other research institutions have specific editions of newspapers in which you are interested. The following are two resources you should consult:

—*American Newspapers, 1821–1936: A Union List of Files Available in the United States and Canada*, Winifred Gregory, ed. (New York: H.W. Wilson, 1937, reprint by Kraus Reprint Corporation, New York, 1967). Your reference librarian should be able to assist you in finding this publication.

—*Newspapers in Microform*, United States, 1948–1983 (Washington, DC: Library of Congress, 1984, 2 vol.). Again, ask your reference librarian to help you find this.

These catalogs are organized alphabetically by state, within each state by town or city, and then by newspaper title. Each entry gives the dates of publication of the newspaper, other titles it may have had, and which research institutions have it. The libraries are listed as abbreviations, which are translated at the front of the volume into names. Some states, such as Wyoming, have their own printed bibliographies, listing all the newspapers that have ever been published within that state.

CHURCH RECORDS

If you still have not found the death certificate or other documents of your ancestors, you may find them in church records. Some church records contain information that cannot be found in other sources, and some provide facts that will support what you have found in other records.

Many churches still have some records, but unfortunately, not all churches that our ancestors attended are still in existence or have records extending beyond more recent years. Even if older records no longer exist, many churches have transcriptions.

If you know the church that certain ancestors attended, try to locate and research the records. Many individual churches still keep their own records. Some of these records have been microfilmed and placed in various collections in the state or are available for rent. The church office personnel can often tell you where the records are available for use.

They can also tell you about denominational universities or archives. Some churches that no longer exist may have given their records to such denominational research institutions in the state or region, local or state historical societies or archives, other local churches of the same denomination, or local public libraries.

Occasionally, historical/genealogical societies and local Daughters of the American Revolution (DAR) chapters know where local church records are kept. Some church records have even been published in historical and genealogical publications.

If you know the ancestor's denomination but not his individual church, try to identify the church from other sources, such as newspaper articles, obituaries, funeral home files, family Bibles, etc. If you have no idea what the ancestor's denomination was, some of these same sources may give you clues. You should also interview some of your older relatives to see if they might know what religious denominations certain family members practiced.

One of the biggest problems with church records is that they are rarely complete. The ministers and priests of individual churches were responsible for recording this information and they were notoriously bad at doing so, particularly prior to the 20th century. It was not uncommon for them to move from town to town; therefore, many early frontier towns completely lacked church records. But if you do stumble across some church records from your ancestors' time, you may find some real gold mines. The diaries of ministers and priests, which are probably the most difficult to find, can contain some of the best information about your ancestors' health and other personal matters. Always inquire if the specific church has a collection of these important documents.

To obtain records from a church that is still in operation, you can either visit the church directly or write to the pastor of the church. If the church of your ancestor no longer exists, you should write either to a local historical society or to the archives of the particular denomination in which you are interested. If they don't possess the records, then they can probably suggest who does. The following churches keep archives:

American Baptist Historical Society
1106 South Goodman Street
Rochester, NY 14620

American Catholic Historical Society
P.O. Box 84
Philadelphia, PA 19105

American Congregational Association
Congregational Library
14 Beacon Street
Boston, MA 02108

Archives of the Greek Orthodox
Archdiocese of North America
10 East 79th Street
New York, NY 10021

Archives of the Moravian Church
41 West Locust Street
Bethlehem, PA 18018

Archives of the Mother Church
The First Church of Christ Scientist
107 Falmouth Street
Boston, MA 02110

Chicago Theological Seminary Hammond Library
5757 South University Avenue
Chicago, IL 60637

Church of Jesus Christ of Latter-Day Saints
Genealogical Association
54 East South Temple Street, Suite 1006
Salt Lake City, UT 84111

Congregational Christian Historical Society
14 Beacon Street
Boston, MA 02108

Lutheran Ministerium of Pennsylvania
Historical Society
Lutheran Theological Seminary
A.R. Wentz Library
Gettysburg, PA 17325

Mennonite Historical Library
Goshen College
Goshen, IN 46526

Presbyterian Church Department of History
P.O. Box 849
Montreat, NC 28757

Princeton Theological Seminary Speer Library
Mercer Street and Library Place
Box 111
Princeton, NY 08542

The Protestant Episcopal Church
Church Historical Society
606 Rathervue Place
P.O. Box 2247
Austin, TX 78768

Union Theological Seminary Burke Library
3041 Broadway at Reinhold Niebuhr Place
New York, NY 10027

Yale University Divinity School Library
409 Prospect Street
New Haven, CT 06520

To familiarize yourself even more with church records, it is advisable to consult the following publications before you proceed:

—*A Survey of American Church Records*, by E. Kay Kirkham (Logan, UT: Everton Publishers, 4th ed., 1978).

—*Religious Archives: An Introduction*, by August R. Suelflow (Chicago, IL: Society of American Archivists, 1980).

—*Directory of Maryland Church Records* by Edna A. Kanely, comp. (Silver Spring, MD: Family Line Publications, 1987).

—*Roman Catholic Church Records and the Genealogist* (National Genealogical Society Quarterly, vol. 74, 271–78).

BAPTISMAL RECORDS

Like birth certificates, baptismal records can provide valuable information about your ancestors' birth and family members. Check with family members to see if there may be copies of these documents in a family Bible or scrapbooks. You'll probably be able to unearth some in your older relatives' attics.

If no family member has a copy, you should first check with an individual church to see if they have your relative's baptismal record in their files. If not, then inquire from them where those records may be—in a local historical society or in the archives of specific church denominations as listed in Appendix D, on page 209.

FUNERAL HOME RECORDS

Funeral homes keep records on the deceased, but they vary in terms of how long they keep these records. Obviously, the files of funeral homes that have gone out of business are likely to have been destroyed. But if you determine which funeral homes handled funeral services for your ancestor, it is worthwhile to try to contact them since their records might be informative.

A good example of the value of funeral home records comes from a genealogist who was trying to learn more about her relative, Maggie Kane Wells of Houston, Texas, who died in 1934. The death certificate listed her birth and death dates and places, cause of death, and the names of the funeral home and cemetery. After the genealogist visited the funeral home, she was handed a file that contained very detailed information about her relative: the color of her eyes and hair, her age, her weight, her height, the cause of death, the names of her children and grandchildren, the name of the cemetery where she was buried with a map showing the plot, and even the fact that she had false teeth!

If you are not sure where the funeral home is located, consult the catalog of the Family History Library under the name of your research locality. If the funeral home is still operating, contact them and try to find out more information.

Getting information about or from records of defunct funeral homes can be challenging. Many such records do not exist, but some do. You should try to determine locally whether the funeral home was sold, who purchased it, and whether the new owners retained the earlier records.

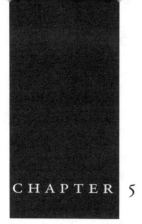

CHAPTER 5

Medical Records

Information about your relatives' medical conditions and illnesses can sometimes be found in hospitals or in the files of insurance companies, and can help you significantly in solving your genetic health puzzle. In most cases, it will be easier to locate the medical records of your more recent ancestors, since the files of most older ancestors have been destroyed or were never maintained.

HOSPITAL AND DOCTORS' RECORDS

Due to patient confidentiality laws, hospital and doctors' records are often not made available even to immediate family members. However, your personal physician can probably obtain copies of them, especially if you discover there are genetic diseases or disorders in your family. The first step is to contact the doctor's office and see what further steps are necessary to obtain the medical records. If your state has strict privacy laws and even your physician can't seem to help, you might want to consider hiring a lawyer to help you obtain them.

Hospital registers will typically tell you the patient's name, age, birthplace, date of admission, illness or disease, and date of discharge or death. Some hospital records, however, are less informative. You can find the names of general hospitals and their addresses and phone numbers in the United States by consulting the National Yellow Book, a directory available in most public libraries. It also lists Veterans' Administration (VA) hospitals and the names of funeral directors.

A death certificate usually gives the name and address of the hospital where a person died (providing the person was in a hospital at the time of death). Using this information, you can then try to obtain the hospital admittance record, which usually contains such vital data as the Social Security number, insurance information and policy numbers, names of relatives, and conventional biographical data. A patient's history will often indicate the number of his or her siblings and the ages of the parents at the time of their death.

Once you have located the hospital where your ancestor died, send your request for information to the hospital's Medical Records Department along with proof of death (a photocopy of the death certificate or even a tombstone photograph) and ask for a copy of the admittance record and patient history. One word of caution! Do not order an entire medical record without first getting an estimate of costs. It could be lengthy and very expensive. If the hospital will not release the records to you directly, enlist the aid of your family doctor.

INSURANCE RECORDS

Insurance company records can be an excellent source of information, including pertinent genealogical facts, such as birth date and birthplace, spouse, and children or other beneficiaries, residence, occupation, death date, and cause of death. If you know a specific insurance company that handled an ancestor's insurance needs, contact them directly for the particular information you need and have not found elsewhere. Usually family records or interviews with older relatives are the best source for determining which insurance company to contact. Your relatives may even have old insurance certificates or other information among family papers that will give you the information you need.

Life insurance records can provide significant information pertaining to the health, age, and lifestyle of your ancestors. As early as 1865, medical information on diseases or health conditions was included on insurance policies. In 1889, Mutual Life began attaching a medical examination to its policy. Since life insurance is usually paid after the death of the insured, the companies kept this information for many years. To protect themselves legally, most companies kept their records long past the death of the insured. These are considered private records and are usually difficult to obtain and find access to. To complicate matters, even though most older insurance companies still exist, they may have a different name. Asking them to search their large files for information on an ancestor can be a useless endeavor.

BECOMING A GENETIC HEALTH SLEUTH

While researching your family health tree, you undoubtedly will encounter terms with which you are unfamiliar; spellings will also vary considerably. Still, you should always record them exactly as you found them in the record. Eventually you can ask your family doctor to translate and explain them to you. Sometimes you can translate them with the help of a medical dictionary and a Latin dictionary. Books have also been published on the history of medicine, which may contain medical glossaries listing terms found in old records.

Here are some of the more common terms you may encounter in older death certificates and other records:

Ague—Usually malaria, but could have been a fever accompanied by chills.

Apoplexy—Stroke.

Bloody flux—Dysentery, shigella, salmonella, amoeba, typhoid, typhus, etc.

Brain fever—Meningitis, encephalitis.

Cholera infantum—Summer diarrhea of infants, which usually occurred the first summer after weaning from breast-feeding.

Debility—Failure to thrive in infancy or old age, or loss of appetite and weight from undiagnosed tuberculosis or cancer.

Dentition—Infantile convulsions, febrile seizures, infected dental cavities, mercury poisoning from teething powders.

Dropsy—Congestive heart failure.

Eclampsia—Convulsions of any cause; later applied more specifically to those related to childbirth.

Hemorrhage and inflammation—Ruptured aneurysm or swollen lymph nodes or superficial cancer with ulceration and bleeding; swollen lymph nodes from chronic infection.

Galloping consumption—Rapidly progressive tuberculosis.

Malignant fever—Fever with hemolysis, malaria with hemorrhagic skin rash, meningococcal infection, putrid malignant fever, or typhoid.

Marasmus and dropsy of the brain—Hydrocephalus and wasting of the body.

Milk leg—Thrombosis in femoral vein, often after childbirth; death from pulmonary embolism or pelvic infection (usual cause for milk leg).

Mortification—Gangrene, usually of the leg, trauma, infection, diabetes, aneurysm of the aorta.

Parisis (paralysis)—Probably from polio, stroke, or syphilis.

Peripneumony—Pneumonia plus pleurisy.

Putrid sore throat—Gangrenous pharyngitis, tonsilitis with peritonsillar or retropharyngeal abscess.

Rose cold—Hay fever (mistakenly thought to be caused by rose pollen).

Softening of the brain—Dementia (syphilitic or nonsyphilitic), cerebral hemorrhage, or stroke.

Stomach trouble—Possibly from complications of gastric ulcer perforation or pancreatitis, hemorrhage, or cancer.

Summer complaint—Diarrhea and vomiting (gastroenteritis).

Most of these records are now in corporation archives, and if you write to their home office, they may aid you in locating the material. But be prepared to show proof of descent from the relative in question and make time to conduct the research yourself. A current agent of the company may also be able to help you gain access to old records, especially if you tell him or her your interest in compiling a family health tree.

For a list of life insurance companies commencing business from the 1800s up to the present, consult *The Source: A Guidebook of American Genealogy,* ed. Arlene Eakle and Johni Cerny (Salt Lake City: Ancestry Pub., 1984). This will provide you with the names, home office, and date of founding for each of the companies listed. Many years ago, some beneficial societies served as insurance providers for members. Many are listed in the Encyclopedia of Associations, which can be found at most libraries. The Family History Library's Record of Benefits, 1883–1924 is a microfilmed resource that might be of help. The original records of this source are at Wright State University in Dayton, Ohio.

Each insurance company handles their records a little differently and they all have different policies regarding requests, so be prepared to spend some time researching this area.

Contemporary medical terms may also be a source of confusion. The major diseases you should be concerned with, since they affect 80% of the population, are heart disease, cancer, and diabetes. The terms used in describing these diseases may be unfamiliar to you, but it won't take long for you to pick up on the most common names.

Cancer terms found on death certificates and medical records come in several categories. The most common names, in general terms, are carcinoma, tumor, malignancy, and metastases (spread of cancer). If a word ends in "oma," it is referring to some form of cancer, such as lymphoma (cancer of the lymph nodes) or melanoma (cancer of the skin). Leukemias are cancers of the blood, such as lymphocytic leukemia and myeloid leukemia. The majority of cancers striking major organs are usually called by the name of the diseased organ, such as lung cancer or kidney cancer. Some cancers have even been named after researchers, which makes it more difficult for you to label, especially when it comes to the more obscure cancers. One of the more common cancers named after a researcher is Hodgkin's disease.

Some of the more commonly used terms for heart-related diseases and conditions contain the root "card" as in myocardial infarction (heart attack) or pericarditis (inflammation of the membrane enclosing the heart).

You may wonder why you have to be so specific in naming types of diseases. When it comes to diseases, the more you know about it, the more you'll understand about its genetic link to you and your family. With cancer, it is critical to be as descriptive as possible in your diagnoses of family members. For instance, if your aunt suffered from breast cancer, was the illness unilateral (one breast) or bilateral (both breasts)? Bilateral cancer tends to be more genetic, so if you find this on your family tree, you should immediately inform your doctor.

Skin cancer is a very loose term for three forms of cancer. The deadliest and believed to be most linked to genetics is melanoma. Basal cell and squamous cell are less serious.

With ovarian cancer, if it started outside the ovary (which happens in 10% of cases), it could be genetic. The stage and grade, which describe the degree and severity of the disease, are also important to know when researching ovarian and other forms of cancer. A higher stage and/or grade usually means a greater chance that the cancer is genetic.

If your relative had colon cancer, it's important to know where the tumor was located (obviously, this can usually only be determined by more recent relatives who were able to explain to others the location). Tumors on the right side or in the cecum (colon) could indicate a bad gene and might increase your own risk.

In general, remember to analyze secondary causes of death as well as primary causes. A death caused by pneumonia, lasting two weeks, is of less significance than an accompanying secondary cause of congestive heart failure.

AMERICAN MEDICAL ASSOCIATION RECORDS

Sometimes trying to locate the records of your relatives' physicians can be challenging. But it can be worth tracking down this information, particularly if the physician is still alive. Since the 1800s, the American Medical Association (AMA) has accumulated information on more than three hundred fifty thousand licensed physicians whose services date as early as 1804. These records are now available on microfilm through the Family History Library. In addition, the AMA also offers researchers a two-volume Directory of Deceased American Physicians: 1804–1929, which provides concise biographical information on more than 149,000 medical practitioners. This resource is available in most large libraries.

FILES OF THE EUGENICS RECORD OFFICE

The Eugenics Record Office (ERO) was created in 1920 to study human genetics and to use this knowledge to reduce genetic problems in humans. ERO researchers set out to create a repository for genetic (including genealogical) information on all human traits. Fieldworkers were trained to go into mental institutions and homes of patients to gather information and document data. It also kept thousands of clippings of marriages and obituaries from major newspapers nationwide. The ERO emphasized the making of pedigrees and the taking of genetic and genealogical information. Recorders noted all afflicted persons whenever two or more people in one family displayed the same disease or condition. In addition to recording extensive pedigrees, the fieldworkers recorded birthplaces and the names of female and male relatives of affected persons.

By the mid-1940s, the ERO lost its funding from the Carnegie Institute. At this point, the records were acquired by the Dight Institute of the University of Minnesota in Minneapolis. These records comprised 18 tons of material, including forty thousand medical pedigrees. Many of the ERO records have been microfilmed and are now available through the Family History Library in Salt Lake City and through its nearly two thousand branch libraries. Because of the nationwide coverage and the enormous number of individuals mentioned in these records, they can be a potentially valuable resource.

As you go through the process of researching medical records on family members, it's a good time to think about your current personal and family medical records. Some day future generations will be trying to obtain information about you and your family. In today's world of managed care, where you run the risk of being juggled from one HMO to another, the state of your medical records is somewhat questionable. If possible, you should get a copy of your own records and keep them in a permanent file at home. Or better yet, there are even personal health diaries, such as *Lifelong: A Personal Health and Medical Journal*, which lets you log your family medical history in a detailed fashion. You can order a copy by writing to *Lifelong*, c/o Irma Cohrs, P.O. Box 7661, Newport Beach, CA 92658.

CHAPTER 6

Libraries and Archives

If you want to be as thorough as possible in developing your family health tree, you will need to spend some time at your local libraries researching your roots. Public, private, and university libraries often own research materials that are invaluable for genealogists and individuals tracing family medical histories.

These collections may include books and periodicals on historical or genealogical subjects, local history collections, vertical files on genealogical information, and specific research materials related to genealogy. Many libraries also have local or regional manuscripts, map and newspaper collections, as well as documents from federal or state governments. Some libraries have a genealogy reference area, staffed with librarians with expertise in this area.

The three research institutions with the largest genealogical collections are the National Archives, the Library of Congress, and the Family History Library in Salt Lake City, Utah. You should, however, be able to accomplish a lot of research in your local libraries before needing access to these national research institutions. Local genealogical and historical societies sometimes have libraries that are open to members and the public at large.

Genealogical and historical societies frequently have computer interest groups (CIGs) that can help you take advantage of what computers and the Internet have to offer individuals tracing family medical histories.

Before you even step foot in a library, however, you should be very clear about what you are researching. It's best if you have already entered some information on your genogram before using resources at a library. Your research will be more productive if you have already answered some of your questions about your ancestors prior to searching for new information. If possible, make your search as specific as possible, such as searching for a birth date or death date.

In general, you should remember the following four points when conducting your research:
- Identify what you know.
- Determine what you want to learn.
- Choose a specific record to search.
- Locate the record and record your findings.

The following major research institutions are well-known for their wealth of genealogical information and other resources:

The National Archives
Pennsylvania Avenue at 8th Street, NW
Washington, DC 20408
(202) 501-5400
http://www.nara.gov

The National Archives and Records Administration (NARA) is known to most Americans as the building in the nation's capital that safeguards and displays the cornerstones of our government: the Declaration of Independence, the Constitution of the United States, and the Bill of Rights. But it is also an independent agency of the executive branch of the U.S. federal government, whose purpose is to select, preserve, and make available to the public historically valuable government records. In addition to its main building in Washington, DC, it has 13 regional branches and 12 presidential libraries.

For some time, genealogists have represented a large group of users of the National Archives, so special efforts have been made to meet their needs. For example, a special free publication, called *Aids for Genealogical Research*, is available by contacting the Publications Department of the National Archives, Room G9. You can phone for this and other publications at (202) 501-7190 or (800) 788-6282.

Many of NARA's resources are also available online at the website listed above. The National Archives also offers genealogy workshops and courses each year. For more information about specific programs, you should contact the number of the regional archives nearest you. (A list of these is provided in Appendix A, on p. 175.)

The Library of Congress
1st-2nd Streets, NW
Washington, DC 20006
http://www.loc.gov

Housed in three buildings in the nation's capital, the Library of Congress is another national research resource for individuals tracing their family histories. The Library of Congress is the home of the largest number of published family histories in the United States, making it a treasure trove of information for the serious genealogist. These thousands of volumes are alphabetized according to family name, making it fairly simple for you to conduct your research.

The major genealogical collection at the Library of Congress is found in the Local History and Genealogy Reading Room on the ground floor of the Thomas Jefferson Building, Room LJ G20. The genealogical collection here has roots that go back to Thomas Jefferson.

One important resource that can acquaint you with what the Library of Congress has available for genealogical research is *The Library of Congress: A Guide to Genealogical and Historical Research*, by James C. Neagles (Ancestry, 1990). The Library of Congress has a very useful website that provides a variety of resources to genealogists. The Library of Congress's catalog can be searched online with LOCIS (Library of Congress Information System).

> Family History Library and Centers
> 35 North West Temple
> Salt Lake City, UT 84150
> (801) 240-2584
> http://www/lds.org/Family_History_Do_I_Begin.html

The Church of Jesus Christ of Latter-Day Saints, abbreviated LDS, maintains the largest genealogical library known to man in Salt Lake City and some twelve hundred branch libraries throughout the world. Every year LDS spends millions on genealogical research, primarily because their doctrine stipulates that all members of the church maintain a thorough and accurate record of their ancestors. You, however, need not be a member of the LDS church to use materials at their Family History Library (FHL). To find the center nearest you, call (800) 346-6044.

Some materials are available on interlibrary loans (see p. 87), and some are not. To acquaint yourself with this enormous library, consult *The Library: A Guide to the LDS Family History Library*, Johni Cerny and Wendy Elliott, eds. (Salt Lake City: Ancestry, 1988).

The FHL has more than 300 thousand volumes and 2 million rolls of microfilm in its collection, and it continues to film original and compiled records from around the world. The FHL Catalog is available on microfiche and on CD-ROM. It tells you which county and state records, censuses, church and cemetery records, and a host of other materials are available on loan or in Salt Lake City. These materials come to the centers on microfilm or microfiche.

Another vital resource is the Ancestral File, on CD-ROM, which is a compilation of descendancy reports, family group sheets, and pedigree charts submitted by church members, nonmembers, and genealogical organizations specifically to this collection, which is updated periodically. Important information is included on birth, marriage and death dates and places, spouses' and children's names, and the names and addresses of those who submitted information.

The main FHL in Salt Lake City and its branch centers are staffed by trained volunteers who can assist you with your search. The best way to obtain resources from the FHL is to make a trip to Salt Lake City. If this is not possible, the next best thing is to visit one of its two hundred branch libraries throughout the U.S. You will not find as much material as in Salt Lake City, but the staff of the regional libraries can always order resources from the main library at a nominal fee.

OTHER SPECIAL LIBRARIES

The following three nationally recognized libraries also have strong collections in genealogy and family history. (See Appendix C, on p. 187, for additional libraries that have special genealogical collections.)

Allen County Public Library
900 Webster Street
Fort Wayne, IN 46802
(219) 424-7241
http://www.acpl.lib.in.us

Newberry Library
60 W. Walton Street
Chicago, IL 60610
(312) 943-9090

New York City Public Library
Local History and Genealogy Division
Fifth Avenue and 42nd Street
New York, NY 10018
(212) 930-0828
http://www.nypl.org/research/chss/lhg/genea.html

INTERLIBRARY LOAN

If your local library does not have the materials you are looking for, there is a good chance that they can be obtained through an interlibrary loan. Reference librarians usually handle requests for interlibrary loans. In asking for an interlibrary loan, you will need to provide the reference librarian with the accurate title, author, publication information, and page numbers, if applicable. Some public or state libraries will loan to other libraries within their own state. Interlibrary loan is also possible through various genealogical and historical institutions.

NATIONAL GENEALOGICAL SOCIETIES

No research about your ancestors would be complete without consulting some of the national genealogical societies in the United States. The following three are known for their resources and expertise in genealogy.

The National Genealogical Society
4527 17th Street North
Arlington, VA 22207
(703) 525-0050
http://www.genealogy.org/~ngs

The National Genealogical Society (NGS) has more than fifteen thousand members throughout the United States. Some of its services include a library and library loan program, a quarterly journal, bimonthly newsletter, home-study courses, annual conferences, and computer interest groups. The NGS website has information for both beginner and advanced genealogists.

> The New England Historic and Genealogical Society
> 101 Newbury Street
> Boston, MA 02166
> (617) 536-5740
> http://www.nehgs.org

Founded in 1854, the New England Historic and Genealogical Society has a library with holdings of more than one hundred fifty volumes and a twenty thousand-volume circulating collection that is available to members.

> The Daughters of the American Revolution
> 1776 D Street, NW
> Washington, DC 20006
> (202) 628-1776
> http://www.ultranet.com/~revolt

The Daughters of the American Revolution (DAR) is a membership society with an excellent library, which is open to the public for a small fee. The library contains a large collection of family histories and cemetery records that have been gathered by local chapters around the country.

LOCAL GENEALOGICAL AND HISTORICAL SOCIETIES

You may want to consider joining your local genealogical or historical society. For a small annual fee, you will have access to magazines, books, libraries, and specialists who can help steer you in the right direction as you develop your family health tree.

Appendix D, on page 209, provides a state-by-state list of the names and addresses of local genealogical societies. You should consider joining one that is near your home or is located near where the majority of your relatives came from.

CHAPTER 7

Creating a Family Health Tree

N ow that you've completed your research, the next step toward understanding your family medical history is to create a family health tree, or genogram—a simple graph that highlights the illnesses and medical conditions of your relatives. To make the genogram most meaningful, it is important to go back at least three or four generations (with a little research, most people can go back at least that far).

Genograms originally developed from research on family systems by Murray Bowen, M.D., a psychiatrist who felt that understanding the relationship patterns of family members could help individuals pinpoint their individual talents, strengths, and weaknesses. Genograms today are also used to graphically display one's family health history, focusing on inherited diseases and medical problems. Once completed, a genogram can give you the "big picture" of your family, both currently and historically.

One fascinating aspect of genograms is that they indicate health and even relationship patterns recurring across generations. For instance, a woman with an alcoholic father may marry an alcoholic herself. Over the years she has developed coping skills to deal with a problem that feels familiar to her; therefore, these skills can be transferred easily to a new relationship, regardless of how destructive alcoholism has been in her life.

A SIMPLE FORMAT

A genogram is relatively easy to develop as long as you stick to the format as shown in Figure 2, on page 94. This design is laid out in such a way to allow you to view both horizontally across immediate family bloodlines and vertically down through the generations. Figure 3, on page 95, gives you the most commonly known symbols used to describe basic family membership and structure. These symbols will help make your genogram uncluttered and easy to read.

As a starting point, your genogram should include the following information about you, your parents, siblings, and grandparents.

- Name, birthdate, and, if deceased, date of death. (The exact date is preferred, but get an approximation if it is not available. This will assist you when ordering a death certificate.)
- Cause of death. (Be as specific as possible. How long did the illness last? Try to get the age of onset of the cause of death.)
- Ethnic background.

- Height and weight.
- Siblings in each generation. Describe birth order (list oldest to youngest, left to right). Note whether there was a large gap—six years or more—between siblings. Chart any deaths, including miscarriages or infant deaths.
- Marital history, including years of marriage, divorces, deaths of spouses, and remarriages.
- Health or psychological problems—chronic illnesses, heart disease, cancer, alcohol or drug abuse, smoking, depression, suicide, eating disorders.

EXPANDING THE GENOGRAM

You have now laid the foundation for your family genogram. Next, it's time to take that same graph and add some aunts, uncles, cousins, adopted children, second marriages, and any other events that could influence your family medical history.

If you're still a little unsure about how to proceed, it might be a good idea to start by writing down all of the information you have gathered about each person on a separate sheet of paper. From that list you can then select the pertinent information that should be recorded on the genogram.

The first thing on your list should be actual diagnosed illnesses and conditions. In some cases, these diagnoses will be very obvious: for example, your uncle who died of a heart attack or your grandmother who developed Alzheimer's disease. But when you go back a little further, it may not be clear which relatives had experienced specific diseases or conditions.

FIGURE 2

A FAMILY GENOGRAM

This genogram covers four generations of a fictitious family. The eight great-grandparents are shown in Generation I; the four grandparents in Generation II; and two parents in Generation III. The male relative in Generation IV, who is compiling the genogram, is shaded. Siblings in each generation may be added. The most commonly used symbols for genograms are listed in Figure 3 on next page.

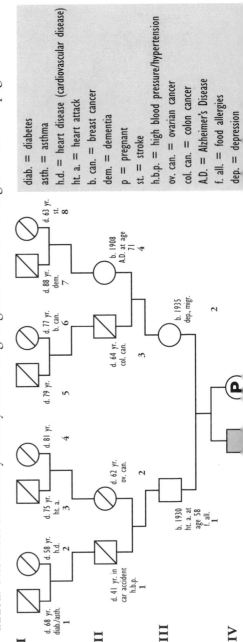

diab. = diabetes
asth. = asthma
h.d. = heart disease (cardiovascular disease)
ht. a. = heart attack
b. can. = breast cancer
dem. = dementia
p = pregnant
st. = stroke
h.b.p. = high blood pressure/hypertension
ov. can. = ovarian cancer
col. can. = colon cancer
A.D. = Alzheimer's Disease
f. all. = food allergies
dep. = depression

FIGURE 3

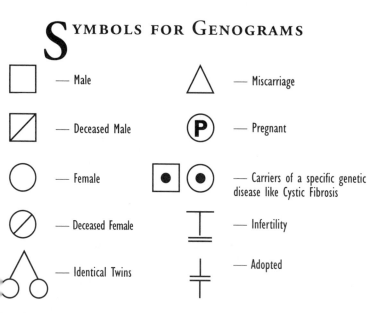

Symbols for Genograms

☐ — Male

◻ (with diagonal) — Deceased Male

◯ — Female

⊘ — Deceased Female

⟨twins⟩ — Identical Twins

△ — Miscarriage

Ⓟ — Pregnant

▣ ⊙ — Carriers of a specific genetic disease like Cystic Fibrosis

⊥ — Infertility

⊥ — Adopted

NOTE: You can modify your genogram by using designated colors or patterns for specific types of diseases. For instance, for types of cancer, you can color in the shapes (■●); for heart disease you can use a patterned design (▤◉).

Occasionally, the death certificates of some of your more distant ancestors may not even give an accurate description of the individual's death. For instance, the cause of death may read dropsy instead of congestive heart disease. Chapter 5 offers tips on how to obtain the appropriate information in these cases.

When you are recording health histories, you don't want to include every cold or flu, but you do want to include illnesses of a chronic or recurring nature, such as sinusitis (nasal infections) or asthma. Obviously, you should include all serious and fatal diseases. Most people who start this process will begin noticing that the illnesses in their families tend to fall into categories. In other words, they will find several people all suffering from heart disease, cancer, or specific psychiatric illnesses.

A CRASH COURSE IN GENETICS

To help you understand more about your own genetically related health risks, you need to understand a little about genes—our body's building blocks. Even if you flunked high school biology, you will be able to grasp the key concepts that make up the framework of medical genetics. The Austrian monk Gregor Mendel, now known as the "Father of Genetics," deduced the basic laws of heredity in the 1860s by studying the breeding of plants and flowers. Despite his discoveries, the molecular basis of heredity remained a total mystery for more than three decades.

Today, information about genetics moves at an ever-increasing pace. Yet the foundation of human genetics is relatively simple and has been known for some time. Each of the billions of cells you are composed of features 46 chromosomes—fast-moving little jellies containing fifty thousand to one hundred thousand submicroscopic blobs, called genes. These chromosomes consist of 23 pairs—one chromosome from your dad and one from your mom. From the moment the first chromosome from the sperm found a matching partner from the egg, your blueprint was created. Your physical appearance—potential height, build, hair color, facial features, eye color—was fully determined. Your sex was established. Your possible talents and abilities were created. Much of your personality and emotional makeup was decided.

But in addition to these unique traits, the potential for specific illnesses or conditions—some trivial and some serious—was also handed down to you.

If you find this type of pattern, it will be very significant, since it will likely indicate a genetic predisposition for those illnesses in your family. By tracing its course over generations, you will probably be able to tell its mode of transmission—whether autosomal dominant, recessive, or X-linked (see pp. 98–102 for more detailed information). Based on the information you obtain regarding your ancestors' environmental influences—such as working in a coal mine or eating a fatty diet—you may also be able to pinpoint multifactorial transmission. In some instances you will even be able to predict who might develop these conditions in present and future generations.

One problem you might run into as you analyze your family's medical past is deciding which illnesses should be grouped together as a category. And if one relative had 10 things wrong with her, how can you fit them all into one genogram? First of all, a list of the most common disease categories is shown in Figure 4, on page 103. Second, if you run into an individual who experienced many different medical problems, it will be helpful if you categorize these specific conditions. In most instances they can be divided up into heart and blood vessel disorders, cancer, respiratory illnesses, neurological problems, etc. By listing a disease as a specific category rather than listing every specific illness, you will have more room on your genogram.

Your genogram will also be clearer if you use simple abbreviations for diseases. For example, imagine trying to fit "agammaglobulinemia" onto your chart! Once you have noted the disease category and given it a simple abbreviation, fill that in next to the individual's symbol on your genogram.

After you have put all your abbreviations into place, here is an important tip: List them somewhere at the bottom of your genogram or on a separate, attached sheet, together with the full names of illnesses they represent. This will ensure that you and your doctor understand exactly what diseases you have recorded.

YOUR UNIQUE BLUEPRINT

How can only 46 chromosomes carry the unbelievable amount of genetic information required to create something as complex as you? The key lies with the extraordinary number of genes that comprise those chromosomes. Genes are nucleic acid molecules that contain a chemical compound called deoxyribonucleic acid, or DNA, as it is more commonly known. DNA gives genes their two most vital abilities: the ability to reproduce themselves and the ability to produce proteins—the organic compounds that are essential to tissue growth.

One of the most amazing things about genes is that each one is unique. Each has a unique chemical effect, which is the reason every human being has their own, individual genetic makeup. But just as genes can determine the color of one's hair or eyes, genes can also be linked to specific diseases or medical conditions. Some of these illnesses are passed along through a single gene, which may be dominant, recessive, or sex-linked. Some genetic disorders result from the interaction between genes with other genes, or genes with environmental factors. This pattern of transmission is called multifactorial inheritance.

Specifically, with the exception of multifactorial inheritance patterns, there are three mechanisms by which genetic defects may be transmitted from one generation to another: 1) autosomal dominant inheritance, in which the trait is inherited from one parent and from the previous generation; 2) recessive inheritance, in which both parents are unaffected; and 3) X-linked (or sex-linked) inheritance, in which the gene for the characteristic is known to be on the X chromosome.

AUTOSOMAL DOMINANT INHERITANCE: WHEN GENES PLAY KING OF THE HILL

Autosomal dominant inheritance occurs when dominant genes have a tendency to overpower those with which they are paired. For example, a gene for brown eyes from one parent will more often than not result in a brown-eyed child, even when the other parent passes down the gene for blue eyes. When a parent has a dominant gene for a disease, there is a 50% risk that each child will manifest the defect, even though it might not be evident at birth. On the other hand, there is an equal likelihood that a child will not receive the abnormal gene; thus, that child and his or her children should be free from the defect. Some of the more than two thousand confirmed or suspected autosomal dominant disorders include: Huntington's disease; hypercholesterolemia (high blood cholesterol levels, with propensity to heart disease); and chronic simple glaucoma.

RECESSIVE INHERITANCE: WHEN BOTH PARENTS ARE THE CARRIERS

Recessive inheritance occurs only if both parents carry the same recessive gene. In most instances, neither parent is aware of being a carrier until the disorder becomes apparent in their child. Recessive inherited diseases tend to be severe and often cause death early in life. When both parents carry a harmful recessive trait, each of the children runs a 25% (or one in four) risk of developing that genetic disease, and each has a 50% chance of receiving only a single defective gene and becoming an outwardly normal carrier of the genetic trait like the parents.

Parents who have one child affected by a disorder due to a recessive inheritance may think that a 25% risk means that the next three children are not endangered. This is not true! The risk of genetic disease is the same for every child of the same mother and father.

Researchers have confirmed more than one thousand suspected autosomal recessive disorders, including cystic fibrosis, galactosemia, phenylketonuria, sickle cell disease, thalassemia, Tay-Sachs disease, and Gaucher disease.

X-LINKED (OR SEX-LINKED) INHERITANCE: WHEN MOTHERS ARE THE CARRIERS

X-linked, also known as sex-linked, inheritance occurs when genes are passed along primarily on the X chromosome that comes from mothers. Normal females have two X chromosomes. Normal males have one X and one Y. In X-linked inheritance, a clinically normal mother carries a faulty gene on one of her X chromosomes. In such a case, each son has a 50-50 risk of inheriting that gene and developing the disorder. Since boys inherit only one X chromosome, unlike their female counterpart, they have no second healthy chromosome to counterbalance the faulty gene.

Each of the mother's daughters has an equal chance of being a carrier like her mother and is usually unaffected by the disease but is capable of transmitting it to her sons. No male-to-male transmission of X-linked disorders can occur. In other words, a father cannot pass the disorder on to his son. Some of the more than two hundred confirmed disorders transmitted by a gene or genes on the X chromosome include hemophilia, color blindness, muscular dystrophy (some forms), and agammaglobulinemia (lack of immunity to infections).

MULTIFACTORIAL INHERITANCE: MORE NATURE THAN NURTURE

Although less defined, multifactorial inheritance occurs when genes interact with other genes, often from both sides of your family, or primarily with environmental factors, such as diet, lifestyle, exposure to drugs, chemicals, or infections. It's important to point out that no one has a perfect collection of genes. Each of us has some mutations in our DNA. In fact, it has been estimated that each of us has about eight genes where changes have occurred that could severely affect our health. Fortunately, though, a change in our DNA does not always show up as a genetic disease or disorder.

With one child in a family being affected by a multifactorial inheritance transmission, chances of other children having the same defect are 5% or less. Although the number of disorders linked to multifactorial inheritance is unknown, some that are thought to be linked include congenital heart defects, cleft palate, cancer, heart disease, Alzheimer's disease, alcoholism, obesity, and diabetes. Many multifactorial inherited conditions, such as alcoholism or obesity, are passed on by a mix of inborn tendencies and family habits, such as the daily martini hour or a love for junk food.

COMMON GENETIC DISORDERS: ARE YOU AT RISK?

For many years, most inherited diseases were believed to surface in childhood. Now it is known that many inherited diseases and conditions occur well into adulthood. Some affect only males, others only females. Some affect each sex. Some genetic disorders are widespread in the population while others only affect certain ethnic or racial groups.

But despite the variation in genetic disorders, the more close relatives who suffered one of the following conditions (and the younger they were at the time), the likelier you are to have inherited a predisposition to that particular illness: heart disease, high blood pressure, diabetes, breast cancer, and colon cancer. These diseases and other less frequent genetic illnesses are covered in more detail in the *Glossary of Genetic Diseases.*

FIGURE 4

Illnesses and Medical Conditions

Cancer

bladder

breast

colon

lung melanoma

neuroblastoma

ovarian

pancreatic cancer

prostate cancer

retinoblastoma

stomach

Cardiovascular

aorta coarctation (narrowing)

aortic aneurysm

arrhythmias (irregular heartbeats)

arteriosclerosis (hardening of arteries)

atrial fibrillation (very rapid heartbeat)

cardiac failure

cardiomyopathy (disease of heart muscle)

coronary artery thrombosis

heart valve failure

high blood pressure/ hypertension

infarction (blockage)— heart, brain, or lungs

ischemia (narrowing of the vessels)

murmurs

myocarditis (inflammation of heart)

pericarditis (inflammation of heart covering)

phlebitis (inflammation of veins)

pulmonary embolism (blood clot in lung)

rheumatic fever

stroke

varicose veins of legs

Respiratory

allergies

asthma

bronchitis

bronchospasm (wheezing)

cystic fibrosis

emphysema

hay fever

laryngitis

respiratory failure

sinusitis

Nerve/Muscle/Bone

achondroplasia (dwarfism)

Alzheimer's disease

amyotrophic lateral
  sclerosis (ALS)

arthritis

back problems

clubfeet

depression/schizophrenia

dislocated hips at birth

dystrophy

fainting spells

learning disabilities

mental retardation

migraine headaches

osteoporosis

seizures/convulsions/epilepsy

speech difficulties

shaking/twitching

tall/short stature

weakness

Gastrointestinal

calculus (stone)—gall
  bladder, kidney

celiac disease

cholecystitis (gall bladder
  inflammation)

cirrhosis

colon disorder

colostomy

diabetes

gall bladder disease

pancreatitis

thyroid/goiter

ulcer/colitis

Reproduction/ Excretion

bladder/kidney infections

hemorrhoids

infertility

miscarriages

prostate problems

undescended testicles

Eye Disorders

astigmatism

blindness

cataracts

color blindness/night blindness

conjunctivitis

different colored eyes

farsighted/nearsighted

glaucoma

retinal detachment/retinal problems

thick glasses/eye surgery/ eye patch

Ear Disorders

hearing loss/deafness/hard of hearing

middle ear infections

unusual shaped ears

Hair/Skin/Teeth Disorders

acne

baldness

birthmarks

dermatitis

eczema/psoriasis

extra/missing/misshapen teeth

lipoma (fat tumor)

moles

rosacea

skin tags

COMPLETING YOUR
GENOGRAM

Now that you have filled in all the pertinent information regarding diagnosed illnesses, you can incorporate other information on symptoms (frequent headaches, skin allergies) and other medical observations (premature baldness, hyperactivity). See Figure 5 on the next page for more of these signs. These symptoms can be instrumental in helping you and your physician determine specific diagnoses of family diseases. They can also shed light on genetic conditions when they are linked with known diagnoses in other family members, when they occur in several people, or when two or more are symptomatic of the same illness.

For example, if you uncovered that several of your relatives had complained of chronic fatigue, on first glance it would not raise a red flag. But if you had other family members with diabetes, the chances are quite high that those fatigue-sufferers also had diabetes. If these individuals had suffered from cataracts or leg amputations, it becomes very likely that they also were diabetics. You personally might not be aware of the link between these conditions and diabetes, but your doctor would understand the connection and would then help advise you on your own health with regard to this possible genetic transmission.

This example shows how you can become a genetic sleuth as you trace your family medical history, especially when you look back several generations for medical information. However, medical records and death certificates have only recently contained specific information about diseases. That means you may have to do a little detective work when looking for information on relatives who died a long time ago.

FIGURE 5

Symptoms and Signs

back pain

baldness

bed wetting

blurred vision

bow legs

bruising

constipation

cough

cramps

deafness

delirium

dizziness

drowsiness

epistaxis (nose bleeds)

exhaustion

fever

gum bleeding

headaches

heartburn

hiccups

hyperactivity

incontinence

insomnia

mood swings

palpitations of the heart

rashes

sleep disturbances

speech abnormalities

stiff neck

swelling of feet

vomiting

weakness

wheezing

INTERPRETING
YOUR FAMILY TREE

By now, some of you will start seeing some interesting patterns in your family health trees. For instance, you might discover that on your father's side most of your ancestors died at a young age of heart-related diseases, whereas on your mother's side cancer was more prevalent but was diagnosed at later ages. Or for some of you lucky genetic detectives, you might find that most of your family died of "old age" or accidental causes.

While interpreting data, it is important to keep in mind the difference between first- and second-degree relatives. First-degree relatives share up to half the same genes. They include brothers, sisters, parents, or children. Second-degree relatives share 1/4 of the same genes. These would be aunts, uncles, and grandparents.

In general, if your family illnesses are spread out randomly across your family tree, it is very unlikely that there is one specific genetic disease that you should be concerned about. You should concentrate on staying healthy by eating a good diet, exercising, not smoking, and seeing your family physician for regular checkups. If, on the other hand, you see certain patterns of genetic illnesses in your genogram, particularly with your first-degree relatives, you should consider seeing a specialist—either a genetic counselor or a specialist in that disease type, such as an oncologist or cardiologist. You should be particularly concerned if a young first- or second-degree relative (under the age of 50) has had an illness usually associated with older people, such as cancer or heart disease.

You definitely should see a specialist if you discover the following: two first-degree relatives with the same type of cancer or one first-degree relative under the age of 50 with cancer or serious heart disease.

After organizing your family health information, it's a natural tendency to start doing some self-diagnosis. Just remember, even though you may think you have a good handle on your own health risks, it is easy to reach the wrong conclusions. Most genetic diseases exist in many forms and the same kind of disease may be inherited in different modes, such as muscular dystrophy. It would be dangerous to think your family has inherited one form when it really has another with a different inheritance transmission. The following chapter offers advice on how to seek professional help once you have completed your family medical history.

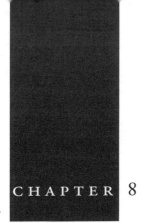

CHAPTER 8

Seeking Professional Help

After completing your family health tree and determining which genetic illnesses and medical conditions exist in your family, you are ready to consult a medical professional. If you see any patterns or "red flags" in your family tree, you should make an appointment with a board-certified physician who is a specialist that treats the disease most prevalent on your family tree. Whether it's a cardiologist, oncologist, neurologist, or other specialist, he or she can address specific questions you have about the disease and can also order appropriate tests on a regular basis for you.

In addition to regular checkups with a physician, you should also consult with a genetics specialist who provides genetic counseling. Often called genetic counselors, these professionals can be found in special units or divisions of many hospitals and medical centers as well as in private practices. These units may be variously named: medical genetics, human genetics, pediatric genetics, clinical genetics, or genetic counseling. Occasionally, genetic specialists are located in clinics that deal with a specific type of condition such as hemophilia or breast cancer. These units typically have a team of health professionals—physicians, researchers, counselors, psychologists, nurses, and social workers—who are all trained in the area of medical genetics.

To locate a genetic counselor, simply ask your primary-care provider or specialist; they can refer you to a genetic counselor in your community. Most major cities have special genetics centers, which are usually associated with a major hospital or medical school. To obtain information on which genetic centers are located in your area, call the toll-free March of Dimes information line at (888) MODIMES.

Another source is state and federal agencies and private organizations that specialize in genetic disorders. For instance, many states have special genetic services coordinators, who can provide information about genetics educational programs, genetics clinics, and genetics support resources. The March of Dimes (listed as a resource in Appendix E, on p. 229) provides a variety of information on birth defects and other genetic disorders. If cancer is the disease you are most concerned about, a free directory of genetic counselors, physicians, and geneticists—who have expertise in counseling about familial risk for cancer—is available through the National Cancer Institute's International Cancer Information Center (1-800-4-CANCER or http://www.cancernet.nci.nih.gov).

The Internet site provides an excellent genetic testing directory, which is searchable by name, city, state, county, and type of cancer or cancer gene.

WHAT GENETIC COUNSELORS DO

Genetic counseling is a relatively new specialty that has grown swiftly in recent years. Most certified genetic counselors in the United States have a master's degree and sometimes a Ph.D. and are certified by the American Board of Medical Genetics or the American Board of Genetic Counseling.

The genetic counselor's major goal is to teach individuals about any possible birth defects and genetic diseases or conditions that may affect their families. Providing information about how heredity works is at the heart of genetic counseling, but good genetic counseling involves even more. Skilled genetic counselors help patients and their families understand the genetic disease or disorder in question, including the accurate diagnosis of the disorder, information about the medical consequences of the problem, and information about the probability that the disorder will occur in other family members. By providing the most accurate, up-to-date information to individuals about these disorders, along with a complete analysis of your genetic history, the genetic counselor can help you make informed decisions about your own or your children's health. A genetic counselor can also advise you about genetic testing and refer you to the appropriate testing center if you desire.

Those most often seeking genetic counseling are pregnant women age 35 or older, because the risk of having babies with certain chromosome defects increases as women reach their mid-30s and 40s. Others seek genetic counseling because they have already had a child with a birth defect or because other family members have a condition or illness suspected of being hereditary. Couples from ethnic groups at high risk of specific hereditary diseases—such as sickle cell anemia in African-Americans, thalassemia in people from Mediterranean countries, or Tay-Sachs disease in Ashkenazi Jews—also look for information.

Genetic counselors use the basic laws governing heredity, as well as the knowledge of frequency of specific birth defects in the population, to predict the probability of the recurrence of a given abnormality in a family.

WHO SHOULD SEEK GENETIC COUNSELING?

Genetic counseling is appropriate for anyone who has questions about their chances of inheriting or passing on a serious genetic disease or disorder. About 10 years ago, genetic counselors primarily saw couples contemplating having a baby or expectant parents. Nowadays, genetic counseling services are becoming more readily available and many different types of individuals seek these services. Here are just some examples of situations where genetic counseling is appropriate:

- An individual has a family history of a known genetic disease.
- A couple has given birth to a previous child with a birth defect or a close relative of the prospective parents has a birth defect.

- A couple has given birth to a child with a chromosome defect.
- An older woman becomes pregnant or wants to become pregnant. (Women age 35 and older are advised to have genetic counseling.)
- One of the parents is, or may be, a carrier of a chromosome abnormality.

WHAT HAPPENS DURING A COUNSELING SESSION?

The genetic counselor will ask you for a copy of your detailed family health tree. During your session, the counselor will address your concerns, summarize the risks, and state specific alternatives. The counselor encourages people to make decisions that reflect their own personal and cultural beliefs, values, and goals. At no point does a genetic counselor tell you what to do, such as having a screening test or whether or not to have a baby. Regardless of their type of training, genetic counselors hold firmly to a professional code that calls for complete neutrality in their work. Throughout the process, you are the ultimate decision maker when it comes to decisions about your own health or whether to have a genetic test.

Those seeking genetic counseling are understandably apprehensive, since the information they may learn could affect their lives dramatically. A good genetic counselor, trained in psycho-social counseling, will be able to ease some of this discomfort and should be able to help you cope with some of the agonizing information that could come out of the session.

To make the most of your visit, start thinking about all the genetic issues affecting you and your family well in advance of the meeting. Write down as many questions as possible to share with the counselor. It is important that you understand everything that is discussed.

When scheduling your appointment, choose the time carefully so that you are alert and don't have any distractions. If you are driving from some distance away, you may even want to consider staying overnight in a hotel in order to have an early-morning appointment when you are fresh.

An appointment normally lasts about an hour. Because many technical terms and explanations are covered, it is essential to make a record of what is being said. This can be accomplished by either taking notes or using a tape recorder so that parts of the session can be reviewed afterward. It can also be beneficial to bring along a relative or close friend who can listen and help you interpret what is being said. Sometimes one person cannot catch all the pertinent facts in one sitting, particularly if they are emotionally involved in the problem.

If at any point during the session the information becomes too complicated or technical, make sure you tell the counselor that you are having difficulty understanding the concepts. Genetic counselors want to hear this type of feedback. Statistical and numerical information can usually be explained in different ways to make it more understandable. A good genetic counselor will also provide you with a written summary of the counseling session as well as brochures about the specific disorder or materials describing genetic tests that are available. Since genetic counseling is usually a short-term arrangement, you should find out before you leave who you should call if you later have additional questions about testing or other genetic matters.

Whatever you do, the point of counseling is to get information, not make impulsive decisions as to whether you should have a child or continue a current pregnancy. Don't expect to find all the answers during a one-hour meeting. Many counselors spend more than one session with people because they know that it takes time to digest information and that new questions may arise based on the increased understanding. You will want to spend some time sorting through the different options available to you.

GENETIC TESTING

During the past 10 years, incredible strides have been made in the area of genetic testing. As scientists continue to identify a growing roster of genetic mutations linked to common diseases, individuals will be faced with major decisions about whether to have or not have a genetic (DNA) test. Before a person can make this decision, they need to have as much information as possible about the nature of the test and its ramifications.

Opportunities for genetic testing are a major topic of discussion during the genetic counseling session. Genetic counselors explain how a particular genetic test is carried out and what it determines. This information would include the accuracy and limitations of the test, the costs and time required and the options that are available once the results are obtained. For some disorders, such as Huntington's disease, there is a defined set of procedures that is followed and the genetic counselor will go over these.

In general, the main reasons for genetic testing include:

- Identifying people at risk of genetic disease who are presently asymptomatic (without symptoms).
- Verifying diagnosis of genetic disease in symptomatic individuals.
- Identifying people who are carriers of a gene that could be transmitted to and cause genetic disease in an offspring.
- Identifying the fetus or newborn with a genetic disease.

Currently, more than one hundred genetic tests are available. While this number may seem large, it is relatively small in comparison to what is anticipated once the entire human genome is revealed. Some of these tests, like the test for Huntington's disease, have been around for some time. Others, like those for breast or ovarian cancer, have been available for only a short time.

TYPES OF GENETIC TESTS

At first glance, genetic tests appear no different than other medical tests, such as tests for strep infections or cholesterol levels. Just as in these tests, the individual undergoing a genetic test provides a blood or some other type of tissue sample from which the genetic material is extracted for examination. The end result is an answer about the state of a particular gene. Genetic tests, however, have some characteristics that greatly distinguish them from regular medical tests. Some genetic tests require the individual to make additional decisions and take other actions before the actual testing can begin. Interpreting the results can also bring complicating factors.

THE DIRECT TEST

A direct genetic test can detect specific mutations or alterations in the DNA of the gene. For an increasing number of single-gene disorders, direct DNA testing is the testing method of choice. The individual seeking the test simply provides blood or a tissue sample and then waits for a brief time for the results. However, in order to interpret the results accurately, it is necessary to know what the exact mutation is. For some diseases, like sickle cell disease, there is only one mutation, so those with the disorder are easily identified by the presence of that characteristic mutation in their DNA. Other diseases—such as neurofibromatosis and some forms of hemophilia—are the result of many different possible gene mutations. In other words, the direct test cannot be used effectively with these because there are so many different possible mutations within the gene that it wouldn't be possible to test for each and every one.

Direct tests for Duchenne muscular dystrophy can detect up to 60% of the mutations; for cystic fibrosis, 90% of the mutations. This means that some people with these disorders will have mutations that the test cannot detect.

THE LINKAGE TEST

Linkage tests are often used when direct tests are not possible. This other approach to genetic testing allows a prediction to be made about the presence of a mutated gene even if there is, at present, no clue at all about what the gene is, what changes have occurred in the DNA sequence or what function the gene serves in the cell. In a linkage test, a region of DNA located near a gene for a disorder is used as a marker, or indicator, for that gene. Linkage testing is more complicated than direct DNA testing because it must first be determined which markers are adjacent to the target genes on both chromosomes. Linkage testing also cannot give an absolutely certain answer about whether a particular gene is present. What it does provide is the likelihood or probability that a particular form of a gene has been inherited along with its marker.

TESTING FOR SUSCEPTIBILITY

One of the newest categories of genetic testing is susceptibility testing, or testing for a gene whose presence can increase the chances of developing a health problem later in life. The important point to remember is that the problem may not develop even if the damaged gene is present, and it may occur even if the gene is absent. Currently the number of susceptibility genes for which testing exists is small, but it continues to grow at a fast pace. Some of the first susceptibility genes found have been for breast cancer, colon cancer, and Alzheimer's disease.

It's important to point out that these illnesses have been shown to occur through a multifactorial, or heterogeneous, transmission. They involve many environmental factors—including diet, lifestyle, exposure to drugs, alcohol, or infections—that interact in complicated ways with the genes in our bodies. For the most part, genes were not solely responsible for these diseases, but they were responsible for tipping the scales so that an individual is predisposed to them. Only

5 to 10% of these genetic illnesses are due to a mutation that is strongly inherited.

Finding that a single susceptibility gene is present does not mean that the corresponding illness will ever develop. This is due to the fact that the susceptibility gene is just one of a number of genetic components that actually contribute to causing the disease. For instance, 15% of women born with a mutant BRCA1 gene will never develop breast or ovarian cancer in their lifetime. Therefore, a factor to consider when deciding whether to have a susceptibility test is the probability of escaping the illness, even if test results reveal the presence of a susceptibility gene.

CARRIER TESTING

Detecting carriers of genetic disease is much more difficult than screening for the disease itself. Because carriers lack the symptoms of the disease, the presence of the defective gene in the individual can be recognized only with special tests. Sometimes, even though the defective gene does not produce symptoms, it may result in a biochemical reaction, which can then be detected.

Biochemical tests for carrier detection are available for only a few genetic diseases. For many genetic diseases, the biochemical basis of the disease is not even known. Another possibility for detecting carriers is by examining the DNA directly. Currently, this is possible for only a handful of genes, because scientists still have no idea where on the chromosomes most disease-causing genes are located.

One disease where carrier testing is available is Tay-Sachs disease. An effective program for screening genetic carriers of the disorder has been developed with the Ashkenazi community—who are primarily at risk for this disorder—and this has led to recent reductions in the number of children born with Tay-Sachs disease. Carrier screening is also available for sickle cell disease, hemophilia, and thalassemia.

PRENATAL SCREENING

The most widespread type of testing for genetic diseases is prenatal screening. Each year in the United States, 4 million women undergo prenatal testing to detect abnormalities caused by genetic mutations. Prenatal screening represents one of the largest areas of genetic screening for two major reasons: 1) Recent advances in technology have greatly improved the way genetic diseases can be diagnosed in unborn babies; and 2) Increasing numbers of women are having babies after the age of 35, when the risk for certain birth defects rises.

Birth defects are generally sorted into four main categories:

- Abnormalities of the chromosomes, such as Down's syndrome.
- Abnormalities caused by alterations in single genes, such as cystic fibrosis.
- Defects caused by environmental factors.
- Multifactorial diseases or conditions that seem to run in families with no clear pattern of inheritance.

Although many genetic diseases are not yet detectable with prenatal testing, the list of those that can be detected is growing at an impressive rate. Most of the tests are highly specific for a particular condition. In other words, each test can detect either one or a few related disorders. Unfortunately, no test can guarantee that a child will be born without any birth defects or medical conditions.

Any couple planning to have children should seek genetic counseling and testing if either of them has a disease with a genetic component, has produced an affected child, or if the mother is 35 or older. Take for example a couple who has a previous child with Hurler syndrome, a metabolic disorder that results in stunted growth, mental retardation, and death usually before age 15. Because this disorder is recessive and the couple has already produced one child with Hurler syndrome, their chance of producing another child with the disease is one in four for each subsequent pregnancy. In the past, most parents faced with this prospect opted for not having any more children. Now, as a result of prenatal diagnostic testing and the option of abortion if the fetus has the disease, many couples in this situation choose to risk another pregnancy. This is a risk worth taking for many of these couples, since they have a 75% chance of having a healthy child.

The most widely used techniques for prenatal testing are ultrasonography, amniocentesis, and chorionic villus sampling (CVS).

ULTRASONOGRAPHY

More commonly known as ultrasound, ultrasonography works a lot like the sonar that allows submarines to see underwater. During an ultrasound, high-frequency sound waves are beamed into the uterus. When these waves encounter dense tissues of fetus, they bounce back. A special instrument then detects the reflected sound waves and transforms them into a picture. By doing this, the doctor can see the fetus inside the uterus without the risk of exposure to X-ray.

An ultrasound, which takes about 15 minutes, is simple and painless. Although the picture produced by the ultrasound is usually unrecognizable to most people, an experienced doctor can measure the size of the baby's head, detect major deformities, and sometimes determine the sex of the baby. Genetic disorders that produce major physical defects, such as dwarfism or hydrocephalus, can sometimes be detected directly with ultrasound. Most of the time, however, ultrasound is combined with other diagnostic procedures, like amniocentesis, to gather more detailed information about the fetus.

AMNIOCENTESIS

Amniocentesis is the most commonly used method for collecting a sample of fetal tissue for chromosome and biochemical analysis. Usually performed during the 16th week of pregnancy, amniocentesis is used to test for birth defects in high-risk women—somebody who has a family history of a genetic disease, chromosomal defects, mental retardation, or is over age 35. During the past several years, early amniocentesis (between 11 and 14 weeks) has also been available for some women.

The procedure, which takes about 15 minutes, is conducted in the doctor's office or an outpatient setting. First, an ultrasound scan is done to determine the position of the fetus. Then a long sterile needle is inserted through the mother's abdominal wall into the amniotic sac, and a small amount of fluid is removed. The cells from the fluid are cultured in a laboratory, which means it usually takes 7–10 days for test results.

Although the test cannot guarantee that the child will be born without birth defects, there are certain conditions that it can rule out, including Down's syndrome, Tay-Sachs disease, amnio acid disorders, and neuro tube disorders, such as spina bifida. It can also determine sex and maturity, and give some indications of general health.

CHORIONIC VILLUS SAMPLING

One of the disadvantages of amniocentesis has been that it is not usually carried out before the 11th week of pregnancy and in some women not until the 16th week. Since only a small number of cells are present in the amniotic fluid at that time, they must be grown in a laboratory for a week or more before sufficient material is available for testing. This means that sometimes the diagnosis is not available until the 18th to 20th week of pregnancy. An abortion performed at this late date poses more complications and is more emotionally traumatic for the parents. This need for a prenatal test that can be performed earlier in pregnancy led to chorionic villus sampling (CVS).

During CVS, a soft plastic tube is inserted through the vagina and cervix into the uterus. Under the guidance of ultrasound, the tip of the tube is placed in contact with the placenta. Suction is then applied to the tube and a small piece of tissue is collected in a syringe at the end of the tube. This tissue, called chorion, contains millions of cells that are actively dividing. Whereas cells obtained from amniocentesis require days before diagnostic tests can be completed, chromosome analysis can be carried out immediately on the chorion cells obtained through CVS. Therefore, if you undergo CVS, you can have results in a matter of hours, compared to the one to three weeks usually required with amniocentesis. CVS can also be performed between the 9th and 11th weeks of pregnancy, considerably earlier than amniocentesis. If an abortion is selected, it can be completed by the 12th week of pregnancy, at a time when complications are less likely to occur and the abortion will be less psychologically stressful to the parents.

ALPHA-FETOPROTEIN TESTING

In recent years, pregnant women have also been offered blood tests for a substance called alpha-fetoprotein, or AFP. Heightened AFP levels in the blood of a pregnant woman can signal that something has gone wrong during fetal development, most often leading to a birth disorder called a neural tube defect. Other markers are analyzed for the possibility of Down's syndrome and another birth defect called trisomy 18.

THE OPTIONS

At the present time it is impossible to cure most birth defects after they have been detected in the womb. However, the information that is obtained through a prenatal test cannot be undervalued. Prenatal testing allows parents to prepare for an unexpected event early in a pregnancy. If parents know ahead of time that their baby will have a particular disorder, they can adjust their lifestyle, meet other families in the same situation, and plan for caregiving. Such plans could include finding out what educational and community programs (see Appendix E, on p. 229) are available for support and reorganizing personal and work schedules to fit the anticipated needs of the new child.

At the same time, individuals will have the opportunity to terminate a pregnancy if careful thought leads them to decide that they do not have the ability to care for a child with extraordinary psychological and medical needs. Few issues evoke as much controversy as does the issue of abortion. But making a decision in which abortion is an option is not like choosing sides between two political candidates. Regardless of whether a person is considered pro-choice or pro-life, contemplating an abortion becomes a very difficult consideration.

TESTING IN NEWBORNS

Genetic testing can also be conducted after birth. This type of screening is done for two reasons: 1) Some genetic diseases are treatable if the disease is detected early; therefore, early knowledge of the disease is clearly beneficial; and 2) Individuals with a family history of a genetic disease are often concerned about whether their child might have the disease with the potential of passing it on to their offspring.

Many genetic diseases can be recognized by specific features right after birth. For instance, infants with Down's syndrome have characteristic facial features that can usually be spotted immediately. Some genetic diseases may require special biochemical tests. Phenylketonuria, commonly known as PKU, is an inherited biochemical disorder that can lead to mental retardation if left untreated in the first few months of life. Because of the severe effects of this disease and because treatment is available, most states and many foreign countries now require testing for PKU soon afterbirth. PKU can be detected by a relatively simple blood test.

GENE THERAPY

For many years, researchers have been working on exploring gene therapy as a way to conquer genetic diseases. The basic premise behind gene therapy is to correct genetic illnesses at their very root by placing the normal gene into the DNA of people who have inherited flawed versions. Restoring the normal genetic makeup would provide people with the capacity to produce the normal protein needed in DNA. Gene therapy has been made possible by allowing a specific gene to be extracted out of the bulk of DNA and to be mass produced or "cloned" in the laboratory. By the end of 1996, nearly two hundred experiments trying out various types of human gene therapy were conducted in the United States.

It is important to remember that as exciting and promising as gene therapy is, it is still in its earliest stages. One of the biggest challenges is being able to introduce the gene into the right cell. A gene for a muscle cell needs to be inserted into a muscle cell, and not into the liver, brain, or elsewhere. Once inside the cell, the gene also needs to work properly. It must direct the production of its protein in the correct amount and at the appropriate time and not in an uncontrolled, erratic fashion. Until these problems are solved, researchers have a long way to go before gene therapy is used as a treatment for inherited diseases like hemophilia and cystic fibrosis.

CHAPTER 9

A Look into the Future

Medical genetics is one of the most exciting areas of science today and is constantly undergoing an incredible explosion of knowledge. Just as early European explorers redrew the map of the world within a few decades of the 15th and 16th centuries, and just as the Russian and American space explorations in the 1950s and 1960s expanded our knowledge of the solar system, today's genetic researchers are making comparable leaps to more clearly understand the human body and heredity more clearly.

As scientists continue to work on creating a detailed map of the entire human gene system, it's just a matter of time before their efforts pay off. Whether it involves improved diagnosis of hereditary diseases or the development of new drugs to help people with these disorders, the results of their research could potentially benefit thousands of people with genetic disorders as well as future generations.

Here are some examples of how individuals can or will benefit from recent developments involving genetic testing and gene identification.

—A woman who is a carrier of the cystic fibrosis gene and wants to have a healthy child could opt for in vitro fertilization, in which several eggs are fertilized in the laboratory and then transferred to a woman's uterus after they have undergone the first few cycles of cell division. When the embryos have grown to consist of eight or 16 nearly identical cells, one cell could be removed and tested in the laboratory for the cystic fibrosis gene. Now the defective gene could be spotted before the embryos are implanted, virtually guaranteeing that this couple's child will be free from the disease.

—Hemophiliacs may soon get what they have long been waiting for: a form of genetic therapy that will repair their flawed gene, which prevents blood from clotting. Researchers hope to begin working with the U.S. Food and Drug Administration on setting up human trials in early 1999.

—Families suffering from a form of hereditary amyotrophic lateral sclerosis (ALS) may some day have access to a treatment as researchers are coming closer to isolating the defective gene. To find the gene involved in causing the disease, scientists at Johns Hopkins University and the University of Pennsylvania studied eight generations of a Maryland family that suffered from ALS by pinpointing afflicted family members and analyzing their DNA samples.

—Researchers at Harvard Medical School recently identified four human genes that may be instrumental in developing cancer treatments with fewer therapeutic side effects. The role these genes play is critical in the area of cell division.

—People with atherosclerotic leg blood vessels may soon be able to avoid bypass surgery as researchers are refining a new gene therapy that restores blood flow in clotted blood vessels. Essentially, the researchers are using gene therapy to grow new blood vessels—a "natural bypass" around blockages in the leg. The gene is injected into the patient's leg, near the obstructed blood vessel. The newly grown blood vessels route blood flow around the obstruction in much the same way that a grafted vessel does.

A BAD SIDE TO GENETIC RESEARCH?

As researchers continue to forge ahead in identifying genes that are linked to the most rare and debilitating diseases or even to conditions as common as baldness or bed wetting in children, it becomes apparent that this information might be perceived as dangerous by some individuals.

One of the concerns being raised by increasing numbers of people is the potential for discrimination. A recent Harvard Medical School study documented two hundred cases of genetic discrimination. One woman was fired from her job as a social worker after her bosses learned that she was at risk of developing Huntington's disease. Civil rights attorneys are concerned that employers who insure their own workers (about 10% of employers), as opposed to signing on with a group plan, may turn down job applicants with a genetic predisposition to various types of cancer and other illnesses that require expensive treatments. Insurance companies could also deny coverage to clients whose medical records indicate that they have a specific genetic illness.

Congress is considering a number of bills that would limit discrimination against people with faulty genes. Some would prevent medical, life, or disability insurers from dropping individuals with positive results or raising their premiums. Others would forbid employers from discriminating in hiring and promoting workers.

Another side to genetic testing that is sometimes overlooked is that despite all the hoopla in the popular press about widespread genetic testing, many individuals who are likely candidates for such testing often do not want to be tested. In addition to fearing that a positive result could lead to a permanent loss of insurance coverage, some individuals feel that they will experience greater stress by knowing that they have a disorder, particularly if there is no effective treatment available at the time. Physicians are also concerned about the accuracy and reliability of many genetic tests. If the tests are wrong, they could lead to incorrect genetic counseling.

Despite these concerns, genetic research is laying the groundwork for novel treatments, involving drug and gene therapies. These new treatments will become major weapons against diseases such as cancer and heart disease.

There is also no question that by gaining knowledge about your own genetic legacy, you will have a greater chance of preventing illnesses. Tracing your roots to learn more about your family medical history can be the most important project you have ever undertaken. When you trace your family medical history, you are protecting the health and longevity of present and future generations.

Glossary of Terms

additive gene—Several genes whose effects combine to determine a trait.

amniocentesis—A procedure, usually carried out at about the 16th week of pregnancy that obtains a sample of the fluid (amniotic fluid) surrounding the fetus. The fluid is collected by insertion of a needle through the mother's abdominal wall and into the sac immediately surrounding the fetus. Studies of the fluid and the fetal cells contained within it can provide information about the fetus's chromosomes, genes, and chemical makeup.

antibody—A protein produced by cells of the immune system that recognizes and destroys foreign substances in the body.

autosomal dominant—A pattern of inheritance attributed to genes located on chromosomes other than the X and Y (sex) chromosomes. The trait or disorder will appear even when only one copy of the gene for that trait or disorder is present. Males and females are equally likely to be affected, and the trait can show up in successive generations of a family.

autosomal recessive—A pattern of inheritance attributed to genes located on chromosomes other than the X and Y (sex) chromosomes. Both copies of the gene in a gene pair must be flawed for a disorder to appear. Males and females are equally likely to be affected. The disorder can appear suddenly with no prior history of it in the family.

autosome—Any chromosome that is not part of the pair of sex chromosomes. Humans have 22 pairs of autosomes, numbered from one to 22.

base—Any one of the four units—adenine (A), guanine (G), thymine (T), and cytosine (C)—found in a DNA molecule.

The order (sequence) of the bases along one strand of the DNA molecule provides information for assembling proteins. The bases on one DNA strand pair up with the bases on the other DNA strand (A with T, G with C), providing stability to the DNA molecule.

cancer—A growth characterized by the presence of cells that multiply and spread in an uncontrollable manner.

carcinogen—A substance that causes cancer.

carrier—An individual who has a gene pair in which one of the genes is flawed. The presence of the flawed gene is masked by the dominant functional gene.

carrier test—A genetic test performed to determine if a healthy individual has a flawed gene which, if expressed in his or her children, could lead to a genetic disorder.

cell—The basic building block of all organisms. The human body is composed of trillions of cells, specialized into many cell types including muscle, nerve, blood, bone, and skin cells.

chorionic villus sampling—A procedure, usually carried out between the ninth and 12th week of pregnancy, to collect cells from placental tissue. Samples can be taken in several ways. Studies of these cells can yield information about fetal chromosomes and genes.

chromosome—A long rod-like structure containing collections of genes. Each chromosome is a long thread of DNA. The standard number of chromosomes in humans is 46.

chromosome mutation—Any change in the number of structure of a chromosome that can be seen under a microscope. Too many or too few chromosomes may be present, a piece of a chromosome may be missing or duplicated, a piece of chromosome may be inverted, or a piece of chromosome may be attached to another chromosome.

collagen—One of the most abundant proteins produced in the human body. It is found in bone, cartilage, skin, and other places that provide structural support.

complex disorder—A disorder attributed to a combination of genetic and environmental factors. Cancer, heart disease, diabetes, and many other common health problems fall into this category. (See also "multifactorial disorder.")

direct test—A test that can detect specific mutations or alterations in the DNA of a gene.

DNA—The abbreviation for deoxyribonucleic acid, the thread-like molecule that is the substance of heredity. DNA has the form of a double-stranded helix. Each strand contains a long sequence of four types of chemical bases (denoted as A, C, G, and T). The sequence of bases makes up the genetic code containing the information for all of the proteins that an organism can produce.

dominant mutation—A mutation whose effect is revealed even when it is present in only one of the genes in the gene pair.

enzyme protein—A type of protein that speeds up or catalyzes a specific chemical reaction. In the absence of the enzyme, the chemical reaction for which the enzyme is responsible will not take place.

exclusion test—A form of genetic test in which fetal cells are examined to see whether they contain the same genetic markers that are present in a grandparent affected with a genetic disorder. That is done when the at-risk parent does not wish to know his or her own genetic status. If the fetus has inherited a marker from the affected grandparent, the fetus will have the same 50% risk of developing a dominant disorder as the at-risk parent. If the marker inherited is derived from the unaffected grandparent, the risk of developing the disorder is much lower.

familial trait—A trait that tends to run in families. It may or may not be influenced by genes.

gamete—A male or female reproductive cell. In the female, an ovum (or egg); in the male, a sperm.

gene—The fundamental unit of heredity; an inherited factor that determines a trait.

gene pair—The two genes, one derived from each parent, with information for producing a protein. One gene comes from the chromosome set contributed by the egg cell; the other gene from the chromosome set contributed by the sperm cell. All genes come in pairs with the exception of genes on the X chromosome in males. Males have only one X chromosome; therefore, the genes on the X chromosome in males are present only in a single dose.

gene therapy—A means of treating or correcting genetic disorders by introducing the normal, functioning gene into the cells in which the gene is defective.

genetic counseling—A multifaceted interaction between a genetic professional and a client in which information about individual and family genetic risks is provided along with related information about tests, treatments, and reproductive options.

genetic heterogeneity—Several different genes producing the same trait.

genogram—A diagram that illustrates the inheritance of a trait in a family over several generations.

genome—The total genetic endowment packaged in the chromosomes; a normal human genome consists of 46 chromosomes.

late-onset disorder—A disorder that is not apparent at birth but develops later in the course of an individual's life.

linkage test—An indirect form of genetic testing in which a known region of DNA located near a gene for a disorder can be used as a "marker"—or indicator—for that gene. This type of testing is used when the target gene has not yet been identified or when a direct test is not practical because the specific mutation is not known.

lipoproteins—Compounds consisting of lipids (fatty substances such as cholesterol) and proteins.

locus—The position that a gene occupies on a chromosome.

marker—A region of the chromosome that can be identified and followed as it is inherited, such as an ABO blood type.

medical genetics—The study of the causes, symptoms, treatments, and prevention of genetic disorders.

multifactorial disorder—A disorder that is brought on by a combination of multiple factors. The contributing factors include several different genes as well as various types of agents from the environment.

multiplex genetic test—A genetic test in which a single blood (or tissue) sample is examined for many different types of mutations.

mutation—Any permanent change or alteration in the number, arrangement, or molecular sequence of a gene.

nucleus—The place within the cell where the chromosomes are contained. It is separated from the rest of the cell by a porous membrane.

prenatal test—A genetic test performed during pregnancy to obtain information about the chromosomes or genes of a fetus.

presymptomatic test—A genetic test performed to determine if a gene (or genes) is present that will bring on a health problem later in an individual's life.

probability—The odds or chance that an event will happen.

protein—A molecule composed of amino acids connected together in a linear fashion. The order (sequence) of the amino acids in a protein is determined by the order of bases found within the DNA of a gene.

recessive mutation—A mutation whose effect is revealed only when it occurs in both genes of a gene pair.

recombinant DNA—Methods for cutting and joining together DNA segments.

sequence—The linear order of the bases in the DNA molecule or of amino acids in a protein molecule.

sex chromosomes—The X and Y chromosomes. Females have two X chromosomes; males have one X and one Y.

single-gene disorder—A disorder that comes about when there is a mutation in a specific gene, and one (for a dominant disorder) or both (for a recessive disorder) of the genes in the gene pair cannot function properly.

susceptibility test—A genetic test for a gene whose presence can increase the chances of developing a future health problem. The problem may not develop even if the damaged gene is present, and it may occur even if the gene is absent.

tumor-suppressor gene—One of a group of genes that functions in the regulation of cell division. If both copies of the same gene are faulty, then an important step in the regulation may be missing, thus contributing to the development of tumors.

X-linked dominant—A pattern of inheritance attributed to genes located on the X chromosome. A disorder will appear when one copy of the gene for that disorder is present. Affected males pass X-linked dominant genes to all of their daughters but none of their sons. Affected females pass X-linked dominant genes, on average, to half of their daughters and half of their sons.

X-linked recessive—A pattern of inheritance attributed to genes located on the X chromosome. Males with the gene will be affected because all the genes on their single X chromosome will be expressed. Females, who have two X chromosomes, can be carriers. Affected males in a family are related through females.

Glossary of Genetic Diseases

When most people think about their health, they are usually concerned about genetic problems that won't affect them. A recent study of women showed that the majority surveyed said they fear cancer most, while only a minority are concerned about having a heart attack. Yet, interestingly, heart attacks are the number-one killer among both men and women in the United States. This same survey showed that of all cancers, women were most afraid of developing breast cancer even though only 4% die from it. Yet lung cancer is the leading cancer killer among women.

The point here is that even though your family medical tree might indicate some rather frightening diseases, it's important that you get as much information about these conditions from your physician, genetic counselor, and other medical resources as possible. Knowledge is power, so the more you know about specific genetic diseases and disorders, the easier it will be for you to make informed decisions about your own health care. In many instances, being knowledgeable about genetics and diseases can also help alleviate some of the fears you may have about your health.

You might be concerned about many similar types of cancer or heart disease that appear in your family health tree. Again, it's important to remember that even though genetics plays a role in your overall health, environmental factors contribute heavily as well. This next section, in which the most common genetic diseases are covered, will illustrate this fact.

HEART DISEASE

Approximately 1.5 million Americans each year have a new or recurrent heart attack. More than five hundred thousand of these individuals end up dying from the heart attack. Heart attacks are just one of many types of cardiovascular, or heart, diseases. In addition to being the number-one killer of both men and women, heart disease has been linked to many genetically based factors—such as blood pressure, cholesterol level and weight—that affect your susceptibility. For this reason, a family health tree can be very useful for identifying people whose relatives had early coronary heart disease and who are likely to benefit from preventive measures.

CORONARY ATHEROSCLEROSIS

Atherosclerosis, which comes from the Greek words athero (meaning gruel or paste) and sclerosis (hardness), involves the progressive narrowing of the arteries that nourish the heart muscle. The narrowing is due to the buildup of fatty plaque along the artery walls. Plaque may partially or totally block the blood's flow through an artery. When this happens, two things can occur: bleeding (hemorrhage) into the plaque or formation of a blood clot (thrombus) on the plaque's surface.

If either of these occur, a heart attack or stroke may result. Atherosclerosis is a slow, progressive disease that may start during childhood. In some people this disease progresses rapidly in their third decade. In others, it doesn't become threatening until they are in their 50s, 60s, or 70s. If your father or grandfather had a heart attack or bypass surgery before age 55 or your mother or grandmother before 65, your risk rises significantly, especially if you are African-American.

Three of the possible causes of atherosclerosis are: 1) elevated levels of cholesterol; 2) elevated levels of triglycerides in the blood; and 3) cigarette smoke or high blood pressure.

HIGH BLOOD PRESSURE

High blood pressure, or hypertension, is defined in an adult as a blood pressure greater than or equal to 140 mm Hg systolic pressure, or greater than or equal to 90 mm Hg diastolic pressure. Blood pressure is measured in millimeters of mercury (mm Hg). High blood pressure can occur in children and adults, but is particularly prevalent in African-Americans, middle-aged and elderly people, obese people, heavy drinkers, and women who are taking oral contraceptives.

If one of your parents has hypertension, your chances of developing it are about 25 to 50%, according to the National Hypertension Association. One of the more recent syndromes that cardiologists have identified is familial dyslipidemic hypertension, defined as a family in which two or more siblings had high blood pressure before age 60 along with blood lipid (fats) abnormalities. Individuals with this condition have a particularly high risk of developing full-blown heart disease.

In large high-risk families, such abnormalities occur at a rate four times higher than in the general population. Even an unrelated spouse has double the risk, perhaps because spouses share the same type of lifestyle.

HYPERLIPIDEMIA

In layman's terms, hyperlipidemia is an elevation of lipids (fats) in the bloodstream. These lipids include cholesterol, cholesterol esters (compounds), phospholipids, and triglycerides. They are transported in the blood as part of large molecules called lipoproteins.

There are three types of hyperlipidemia:
- *hyperlipoproteinemia*—elevated plasma lipoproteins
- *hypercholesterolemia*—elevated levels of cholesterol
- *hypertriglyceridemia*—elevated levels of serum triglycerides

Hypercholesterolemia is the most common form and appears to be caused by both genetic and environmental factors. Cholesterol comes from two sources: 1) it's produced in your body; and 2) it's found in foods that come from animals, such as meats, poultry, fish, seafood, and dairy products. Saturated fatty acids are the chief culprit in raising blood cholesterol, which increases your risk of heart disease.

Familial hypercholesterolemia, which is caused by skyrocketing cholesterol levels, strikes about one out of every five hundred people. Although often underdiagnosed and undertreated, familial hypercholesterolemia is a very treatable condition.

PREVENTION OF HEART DISEASE

Do you feel a death sentence staring down upon you as you scan your family medical tree with all its heart disease-related red flags? Relax. Since heart disease is a unique blend of genetic and environmental (or lifestyle) factors, you need to be very careful in assessing your own risk of developing it. If there was no smoking, heavy drinking, or obesity among your relatives, it is very likely that the heart disease in your family is genetic. However, if there was heavy smoking, heaving drinking, and obesity, along with family heart disease, it will be more difficult for you to assess the strength of the genetic connection.

When it comes to heart disease, whether it is a genetic predisposition or environmental factors, a recurring pattern within your family should be a warning to you to check with your doctor about what lifestyle changes could minimize your risks.

If your cholesterol is over 240, you need to have your blood analyzed for LDL, or "bad" cholesterol. An LDL level over 160 will likely prompt your doctor to prescribe cholesterol-lowering drugs, a restricted diet, and regular exercise. If you are hypertensive, your doctor may advise you to cut down on salt or to take calcium supplements or blood pressure drugs.

One of the most effective strategies in preventing heart disease is to decrease your intake of fat. The American Heart Association advises limiting fat to no more than 30% of the total calories you consume, with less than 10% coming from saturated fats (animal fats like cheese and meat and tropical oils like coconut).

If you have a higher-than-average risk, the American Heart Association recommends that you keep your daily saturated fat intake at less than 7% and limit your cholesterol intake to 200 mg a day. Total fat should not exceed 15% of your daily calories. You should, however, eat fatty fish—like salmon, tuna, mackerel, and herring—since research shows that fish oils are actually good for the heart. In addition, you should limit your alcohol consumption to two drinks a day and don't smoke—it doubles or triples your chances of having a heart attack.

Your physician will tell you how often to have your blood pressure and cholesterol levels checked. Your physician should also advise you on the type of exercise program you should maintain, particularly how much in the way of aerobics you should include, since even though aerobic exercise lowers heart-disease risk, it also puts added strain on the heart.

Women after menopause should ask their doctors about taking hormone-replacement therapy (HRT). In some instances, it has been shown to cut the risk of a heart attack by as much as one-half. Some doctors also recommend aspirin therapy, since regular low doses of this common drug have been reported to lower heart disease risks in some people.

DIABETES

Researchers have established that one's chances of developing type 2, or noninsulin dependent diabetes (the most common form of diabetes) is substantially increased if one or both parents have this type. If one or more grandparents had type 2 diabetes, or a brother or sister has it, you are also at higher risk. Some researchers have said that having one parent with type 2 diabetes increases your risk three-to-four times higher than average. In the United States, diabetes is most likely to strike non-Caucasian ethnic groups.

However, just like heart disease, even if there is a pre-disposition of type 2 diabetes in your family, you will not necessarily contract the disease. Following a healthy diet, controlling your weight, and exercising regularly all seem to help keep the genetic component at bay.

Type 2 diabetes develops very slowly; in fact, some 8 million Americans remain undiagnosed with it. Most people who get type 2 diabetes have increased thirst and an increased need to urinate. Many also feel edgy, tired, and nauseous. Some people have an increased appetite but actually lose weight. Other signs and symptoms include hard-to-heal infections of the gum, skin, vagina, or bladder; blurred vision; tingling or loss of feeling in the hands or feet; and dry, itchy skin. Some complications that are related to diabetes are kidney failure, blindness, and heart disease.

Surprisingly, the type of diabetes that usually starts during childhood, called type 1 or insulin-dependent, does not have the genetic link that type 2 does. Individuals with type 1 diabetes need daily injections of the hormone insulin to stay alive. Only about 10% of all people with diabetes have this form of the disease.

CONTROL AND PREVENTION

The key to staying healthy with diabetes is to control your blood glucose levels so that they are as near to normal nondiabetic levels as possible. This can be accomplished through regular exercise and a healthy diet. Sometimes this is all one needs to do to keep their diabetes in check. Others may need diabetes pills or insulin shots. Individuals who are overweight are advised to lose weight, which sometimes brings their blood sugar levels into the normal range.

If you currently don't have diabetes but many of your first-degree relatives do, you should also follow a healthy diet, control your weight, and exercise regularly. This may be your best insurance against getting diabetes. Based on a study of Japanese smokers, in which men who smoked 16 cigarettes or more a day tripled their diabetes risk, avoiding cigarettes may be one way to help reduce your diabetes risk and curb complications if you have the disease.

CANCER

Several types of cancer, such as retinoblastomas (eye tumors) and colon cancer in families with polyposis (colon polyps that often become malignant) are known to be inherited. Scientists also believe that other forms of cancer run in families, such as cancer of the stomach, endometrium (uterine lining), lung, colon, bladder, breast, and skin (melanoma).

A good physician specializing in cancer and genetics or a genetics counselor can tell you if your family's cancers are hereditary. For instance, if retinoblastomas are present, they are known to be hereditary in an autosomal dominant fashion. If there is just one isolated case, it could be just a fluke, but if there are several cases and they form an autosomal dominant pattern, it's very likely they are hereditary. A genetic counselor can then look at your family tree and determine who in your family has a 50% chance of getting them.

There are also some autosomal recessive cancers that strike families, such as neuroblastomas (cancers of the adrenal gland), xeroderma pigmentosum (a rare but deadly kind of skin cancer), and some brain tumors. Autosomal recessive cancers are less common, since both parents must carry matching recessive genes for them to occur. Even when they do, only 25% of the couple's children will be affected.

BREAST AND OVARIAN CANCER

Nowadays, you cannot pick up a newspaper or magazine without reading breaking news about the genetic connection to breast cancer. Some 5 to 10% of all breast cancers are inherited and at least two of the genes linked to these hereditary cancers have been identified: BRCA1 and BRCA2. Now scientists have found a possible new breast cancer gene, called BAP1, which is also linked with lung cancer.

If your mother, sister, and daughter developed breast cancer before menopause, especially if both breasts were affected, your own risk is significantly higher. If you've inherited one of the so-called BRCA1 or BRCA2 gene mutations, you have—at most—a 55 to 85% chance of getting breast cancer. Your own ovarian-cancer risk is also higher than average. Still, it's important to note that these risks are based on very special cancer-prone families.

Breast cancer is the most commonly diagnosed form of cancer, except for cancers of the skin, and the second most common cause of cancer death for American women. Each year, more than one hundred eighty thousand women are diagnosed with breast cancer. Women who have inherited the gene alterations usually have an increased risk of developing breast cancer at a younger age (before menopause), and they often have multiple family members with the disease. Research has also proved that Ashkenazi Jews (those of Eastern European descent) have a greater likelihood of having two specific alterations in BRCA1 and one in BRCA 2.

Researchers have known for a long time that genetics plays a role in ovarian cancer. If your mother had ovarian cancer, you have an increased risk of ovarian cancer, but if both your mother and aunt have had ovarian cancer, your risk is even higher. Breast cancer can also be an important predictor of ovarian cancer. Many women who have had two or more relatives with ovarian cancer and who have already had children sometimes consider having their ovaries removed to avoid getting ovarian cancer. Although much less common than breast cancer, ovarian cancer is diagnosed in more than twenty-five thousand women every year. During this same time period, about fifteen thousand will die from it.

One of the problems with ovarian cancer, also known as the "silent killer," is that early symptoms, when they occur at all, may be easily dismissed as indigestion or some other minor problem. Tumors, therefore, can spread or grow dangerously large before a woman has any idea something is seriously wrong. Symptoms include pelvic discomfort, bloating, gas, back pain, fever, and abnormal vaginal bleeding. Whether or not you have a family history of ovarian cancer, if you start experiencing these symptoms, see your doctor immediately.

LOWERING YOUR RISK OF GETTING BREAST AND OVARIAN CANCER

While there are no proven ways to prevent breast cancer, studies suggest that there are ways to minimize your chances of getting it. Staying slim, quitting smoking, exercising at least four hours a week, eating a high-fiber diet, and keeping your alcohol consumption down (fewer than three drinks a week) may reduce your risk. You should also do a monthly breast self-exam and have a physician examine your breasts annually, or even more often if you are at increased risk. Check with your physician about having yearly mammograms beginning at age 40 instead of 50.

Eating a low-fat, high-fiber diet may also help prevent ovarian cancer. Some physicians recommend taking oral contraceptives, since they prevent ovulation and may lower the risk of ovarian cancer. If you have a family history of ovarian cancer, regular pelvic exams are critical, once or even twice a year. You should also ask your doctor about regular ultrasound screenings.

COLON CANCER

Researchers have proven that some colon cancers are inherited. John Hopkins University researchers recently discovered a new type of genetic mutation, which may increase the risk of colon cancer. About 6% of Ashkenazi Jews (those of Eastern European descent) are believed to have this gene alteration. This newly identified mutation is believed to confer a lifetime risk of colorectal cancer of roughly 20%— double the normal danger. Genetic tests have recently been made available for individuals who suspect they may have this aberrant gene.

Test advocates believe people who find they have the mutation might be especially motivated to get regular colon exams to check for precancerous polyps. Still, even those who test negative for this mutation cannot rest easy, because most hereditary colon cancers appear to be caused by other genetic errors. If you have a history of colon cancer, you should have regular screening tests (such as a rectal examination, proctoscopy, and colonoscopy) starting at age 35. Colonoscopy is particularly important since it examines the whole colon. Two-thirds of all hereditary colon cancers are found in the upper colon—the part not checked by sigmoidoscopy. Regular low doses of aspirin may offer protection, as does a low-fat, high-fiber diet.

MALIGNANT MELANOMA

Malignant melanoma causes 75 to 85% of skin-cancer related deaths. It is the fastest growing of the cancers and will soon affect nine out of every one hundred persons in their lifetime. People with red hair and fair skin, especially when exposed to excessive sunlight, have been found to be prime candidates for skin cancer. During the past five years, research has shown that about 5 to 10% of melanoma has a strong genetic link. One physical trait that has been found in people with melanoma are irregular-shaped moles called dysplastic nevus syndrome, which are inherited as an autosomal dominant trait. Doctors now know that these moles often turn malignant.

If you have a family history of melanoma or if you have any of these larger-than-normal moles, you should consult with a dermatologist to see if they should be removed. If you sunburn easily and severely, or have a light complexion with light-colored eyes, you should limit your exposure to sun and always wear sun block.

PROSTATE CANCER

Approximately 9% of prostate cancer cases result from inheritance of mutated prostate cancer susceptibility genes. In the United States, prostate cancer is the most common cancer among men, after skin cancers. Signs and symptoms of prostate cancer include difficulty starting and maintaining a flow of urine, pain on urination, having to urinate more frequently than usual, and frequent nighttime urination.

If your family health tree shows frequent cases of prostate cancer among family members, you should have regular screenings beginning at age 40. If your family members had prostate cancer at younger ages with higher-grade tumors, you should ask your doctor about being seen earlier for regular checkups.

NEUROLOGICAL ILLNESSES AND DISORDERS

As the command center for the entire body, the nervous system regulates and coordinates all body functions by continuously reacting to both internal and external environments. The structures of the nervous system are the brain, the spinal cord, and the nerves. Some of the major hereditary diseases and disorders that affect the nervous system are described below.

ALZHEIMER'S DISEASE

In the past few years, there has been a lot of discussion about the genetic link to Alzheimer's disease, a progressive degenerative disorder resulting in continual mental deterioration that cannot be stopped or reversed. Current research proves that about 5% of Alzheimer's disease cases are due to hereditary factors. A test is now available that can detect whether an individual has the flawed gene for Alzheimer's disease.

Alzheimer's disease occurs in two distinct groups of people. More commonly, the disease strikes those individuals in their 70s and 80s, causing a variety of symptoms: memory loss, speech problems, deterioration of intellectual functions, and personality changes. In the second group, patients develop these symptoms at a much earlier age, usually in their 50s or early 60s. Those in this group may have an autosomal dominant form of the disease or they may have inherited a susceptibility to Alzheimer's disease when exposed to certain environmental factors. It is unknown whether a single gene or a group of genes causes familial Alzheimer's disease.

Unfortunately, there is no cure for Alzheimer's disease. In fact, the only way to confirm the diagnosis is by brain biopsy or by autopsy after death. However, during the past few years many medications have been introduced for patients with mild or moderate Alzheimer's disease. If you have traced your family medical history and have learned about some relatives that have suffered from Alzheimer's disease, remember that early-onset Alzheimer's disease is the only version currently being linked to genetics.

AMYOTROPHIC LATERAL SCLEROSIS (ALS)

Also known as Lou Gehrig's disease, amyotrophic lateral sclerosis (ALS) is an irreversible, progressive disease that results in continuous destruction of muscle neurons within the spinal cord and the lower brain stem. The most common form of ALS is known as "sporadic" and may affect anyone. Only about 5 to 10% of ALS cases are hereditary, and the gene responsible was only recently identified. In those families, there is a 50% chance the offspring will have the disease.

More than five thousand people in the U.S. are newly diagnosed with ALS each year. The incidence of ALS is five times higher than Huntington's disease and about equal to multiple sclerosis. Present treatment of ALS is symptomatic relief, prevention of complications, and maintenance of optimal function and quality of life.

GAUCHER DISEASE

Gaucher disease is the most prevalent Jewish genetic disease, occurring in one out of every thirteen hundred Ashkenazi Jews of Eastern and Central European ancestry. Gaucher disease is an inherited "storage" disorder resulting from the deficiency of a certain enzyme. There are three versions of the disease which are distinguished by the absence or presence and severity of neurologic complications. Recently, the gene for the enzyme was isolated and five different lesions in the gene that cause Type 1 Gaucher disease in Ashkenazi Jews have been identified. This now allows for the diagnosis of affected individuals as well as prenatal diagnosis of affected fetuses through prenatal screening.

If one parent is a carrier of Gaucher disease and the other parent is not, there is a 50% chance of having a child who inherits the Gaucher gene from the carrier parent and becomes a carrier of the disease. None of the children will have Gaucher disease because they will have one normal gene inherited from the other parent.

If both parents are carriers of Gaucher disease, with each pregnancy there is a 25% chance of having a child who inherits one Gaucher gene from each parent and thus has Gaucher disease. It must be emphasized that the odds for having a child inherit Gaucher disease are totally independent of whether or not a previous child has the disease.

Because Gaucher disease is a genetic disorder, all close blood relatives of patients are at risk of having the disease, or are potential carriers of the gene. Families with a history of Gaucher disease may want to discuss the possibility of genetic testing with their physicians.

Until recently, patient care and therapy for Gaucher disease was directed at managing symptoms using bed rest, nonaspirin analgesics and anti-inflammatories for chronic pain. Recently progress has been made in the development of safe and effective techniques that promise to go beyond management of symptoms caused by the accumulation of Gaucher cells. The technique involves supplementing or replacing the missing enzyme in patients with the disease. Currently, research is underway that someday may lead to a cure for Gaucher disease.

HUNTINGTON'S DISEASE (HD)

Huntington's disease is a hereditary brain disorder that affects movement, mood, cognitive ability, and emotional control. Caused by an autosomal dominant gene, Huntington's disease usually appears between the ages of 30 and 45. Virtually all affected individuals inherit the gene from one of their parents. However, some parents may die of other causes before the symptoms of Huntington's disease are present, so not all people with the illness know that they had a parent who had Huntington's disease. An individual with Huntington's disease has a 50% chance of passing the disease on to each of his or her children.

One of the unfortunate aspects of Huntington's disease is that because it occurs relatively late in life, many affected individuals bear children before they are aware that they have the disorder. As a result, the disease is easily transmitted from one generation to the next. Interestingly, of the tens of thousands of people in the world who have Huntington's disease, almost all may be distantly related to a common ancestor who first had the disorder several hundred years ago.

Although there is no cure for Huntington's disease, medications can be effective in treating symptoms such as depression and anxiety. In some cases, however, people with Huntington's disease do better when medication is kept to a minimum.

MULTIPLE SCLEROSIS (MS)

As this book was going to press, researchers were studying the possible genetic effects of multiple sclerosis (MS), a degenerative disease that affects the brain and spinal cord and interferes with muscle strength and movement. Many researchers believe MS is related to both genetic and environmental factors; for example, an inherited defect in the body's immune system does not become apparent until it is triggered by a specific virus. MS cannot be cured or prevented at this time.

NEUROFIBROMATOSIS (NF1)

Also called von Recklinghausen disease, neurofibromatosis (NF1) is a genetic disease that causes multiple tumors in the tissue of the nervous system. Occurring in one out of every three thousand births, NF1 is transmitted through an autosomal dominant inheritance pattern. It affects both males and females in all races and ethnic groups. NF1 has no cure. Surgical removal of the growths may be necessary if the eyes or ears are involved. Many individuals have growths removed for cosmetic reasons.

PARKINSON'S DISEASE

Although some families appear to have a higher incidence of Parkinson's disease, a genetic susceptibility has still not been proven. Some researchers believe that a multifactorial cause, in which heredity is combined with environmental causes such as a virus, may be responsible for Parkinson's disease, which often results in hand and foot tremors, forward-slumping posture, and rigid muscle tone. The symptoms of Parkinson's disease can be reduced significantly with medication and physical therapy.

TAY-SACHS DISEASE

This is the most well-known of the Jewish genetic diseases and is an autosomal recessive disorder, potentially afflicting about one out of every twenty-five hundred Ashkenazi Jewish newborns. Children only develop the disease if both of their parents carry a defective gene for hexosaminidase A. Because the frequency of the gene for Tay-Sachs disease is so low in the general population, the chance of two parents carrying a defective gene is remote. However, among Ashkenazi Jews in the United States, about one in 30 individuals carries a defective gene for Tay-Sachs disease. Thus, if two Ashkenazi Jews marry, there is a higher risk that their children will inherit two defective copies of the gene and will end up with Tay-Sachs disease. The infantile-onset version of the disease, which is the most common form of the disorder, causes severe mental and developmental retardation. Death usually occurs within five to eight years of life.

Screening programs for Tay-Sachs disease carriers in the Ashkenazi community have been very successful. The success of this effort is proven by the fact that the incidence of Tay-Sachs disease has declined significantly in recent years.

TOURETTE SYNDROME

Generally classified as a tic disorder, Tourette syndrome is thought to be transmitted through an autosomal dominant inheritance pattern with varying degrees of severity. This variation in symptoms has been explained in part by the fact that environmental factors also play a role in determining the nature of the symptoms, which include uncontrolled, recurrent twitching of the face, head, and shoulders with shouting episodes and obsessive-compulsive behavior. Tourette syndrome is not life-threatening and can usually be controlled through medication or behavioral therapy.

MENTAL ILLNESSES AND BEHAVIORAL CONDITIONS

Researchers are not always in agreement about what is the exact cause of mental illness. For the most part, theories focus on biological, psychological, behavioral, and social-interpersonal factors. It is a fact that some mental illnesses tend to run in families. Whether this occurs because of genetic transmission of a mental illness or because certain behaviors are learned from family members who have mental disorders is still not known. In the near future, it's likely that researchers will uncover genetic markers for many of the mental illnesses that we long ago thought were clearly environmental. Here are some of the more common mental illnesses and behavioral conditions that appear to have genetic links.

ALCOHOLISM

About 10 million people in the United States are problem drinkers, and some 6 million are severely addicted to alcohol. The observation that alcoholism tends to run in families is a very old one, but recent studies have made it possible to know whether these familial clusters are due to genetics, environment, or both. Research by the National Institute of Alcohol Abuse and Alcoholism has provided evidence that both hereditary and environmental factors are involved in many cases of alcoholism.

Researchers have found that 13 to 25% of children of alcoholics are likely to become alcoholics. Alcoholism does not appear to be inherited as a simple genetic trait; it exhibits none of the characteristic signs of dominant, recessive, or

X-linked factors. Alcohol dependence is determined by complex interactions among many genes, and the genes involved also interact with environmental influences.

Even if your family health tree is filled with alcoholic relatives, you should remember that the majority of individuals with a genetic predisposition to alcoholism never become alcoholics and many of those that do become alcoholics are able to overcome this problem. If you suspect that you have a drinking problem, your physician will refer you to the appropriate community programs that can help with your problem.

ANXIETY DISORDERS

For many years, researchers have speculated that anxiety disorders, such as obsessive-compulsive disorder, panic disorder, and phobic disorder, tend to run in families. These disorders have also been linked to certain medical conditions, such as thyroid gland and adrenal gland abnormalities or chemical substance intoxication. Depending on the specific anxiety disorder, treatment may include individual, group and/or family therapy; relaxation techniques; behavior modification; or medication.

ATTENTION DEFICIT DISORDER

Today it is widely accepted that a genetic component is linked to the mixture of behaviors that characterize attention deficit/hyperactivity disorder (AD/HD), a condition marked by hyperactivity, impulsive behavior, and an inability to focus or pay attention. Attention deficit disorder is considered a learning disability, which means if it goes undetected, affected children can suffer from frustration, shame, and low self-esteem.

If diagnosed correctly, attention deficit disorder can be successfully treated with medication or behavioral modification.

EATING DISORDERS

The two eating disorders—anorexia nervosa and bulimia—have long been known to run in families. Anorexia nervosa is a disorder characterized by obsessive fear of becoming fat. Twin studies have indicated that two identical twins are more likely to both have anorexia than are two nonidentical twins, which supports the theory that genes influence the disease. Bulimia involves the rapid consumption of large amounts of food over a short period of time, usually in less than two hours. The binging episode usually ends when abdominal pain or self-induced vomiting occurs. A number of studies indicate that close relatives of bulimics tend to have higher than expected rates of depression.

MANIC DEPRESSION (BIPOLAR DISORDER)

Researchers agree that manic depression has a strong genetic influence, but they disagree over its mode of inheritance. Some claim it's a simple mode of inheritance, such as autosomal dominant or X-linked dominant. Others have suggested that the disease displays a complex pattern of inheritance, resulting from the interaction of many genes as well as environmental factors. Not everyone with a vulnerable genetic makeup will develop depression and some people believe stress often triggers its onset.

Cognitive therapy is very effective in teaching methods for combating the negative thought patterns that contribute to depression. A physician will typically refer a patient suffering from signs of depression to a mental-health professional. By seeking help when mild symptoms appear, an individual suffering from depression can sometimes avoid a full-blown attack. Exercise programs and antidepressant medications can also help.

SCHIZOPHRENIA

Schizophrenia produces a variety of symptoms (delusions, hallucinations, confused thinking)—none of which are present in all schizophrenics. The word "schizophrenia" means "split head," and the disease is mistakenly thought of as "split personality." However, it does not involve multiple personalities and should not be confused with multiple personality disorder. Many studies over the years have consistently demonstrated that schizophrenia tends to run in families. If one parent has schizophrenia, his or her child has about a 10% chance of developing the disease. If both parents have schizophrenia, each of their children has about a 40% chance of becoming schizophrenic. However, it is important to point out that the observation that schizophrenia runs in families does not prove that the disease is hereditary. A number of members of a family may be schizophrenics because of predisposing environmental factors they share.

In spite of strong evidence that genes are responsible for schizophrenia—through studies of identical twins and adopted children whose biological parents were schizophrenics—

the exact mode of inheritance is still unproven. Researchers have suggested three different ways. Some feel it results from a major gene that produces a predisposition to the disorder. This gene would be inherited in a simple way, perhaps as an autosomal dominant trait. However, not everyone who inherits this gene would develop schizophrenia, since environmental factors sometimes come into play. Other geneticists think that schizophrenia arises from the interaction of many genes and environmental factors, or in a multifactorial transmission. The third suggestion is that schizophrenia is not a single disease, but several separate diseases that only appear similar.

Treatment for schizophrenia includes antipsychotic medication, individual or group therapy, social skills training, and hospitalization.

OTHER GENETIC DISEASES

CLEFT LIP AND CLEFT PALATE

Sometimes called a hair lip, cleft lip is a notch or vertical split in the upper lip. The cleft may be only partial or it may extend all the way up to the base of the nose. Cleft lip is often accompanied by cleft palate, which is a split that runs down the roof of the mouth. Most often cleft lip and cleft palate, which occurs in approximately one out of every 930 births, exhibits multifactorial inheritance, meaning that a number of genes and environmental factors interact to produce the disorder. If parents without clefts have a child with a cleft, the chance that a subsequent baby will have a cleft is 2 to 4%.

While little is known about how to prevent cleft lip and palate, a recent study shows that taking multivitamins containing folic acid before conception and during the first two months of pregnancy may help prevent them. Other studies have shown that fetuses with a certain predisposing gene may be at increased risk of developing cleft palate if their mothers smoke. In addition, other factors, such as maternal alcohol abuse, maternal diabetes and some types of medications have been linked to increased risk of cleft palate. Preventive measures include avoiding alcohol and tobacco during pregnancy, maintaining good control of diabetes before and during pregnancy, using only medications prescribed by a physician who knows of the pregnancy, and getting early and regular prenatal care.

CLUBFOOT

Clubfoot is a relatively common birth defect characterized by a foot that is twisted out of its normal position. Clubfoot occurs in about one out of every 735 births in the general population. Recent studies of the inheritance of clubfoot suggest that the deformity results from the influence of both a major dominant gene and multifactorial effects. If two normal parents have a child with clubfoot, the risk of having another child with clubfoot is 3%. If one parent has clubfoot, the risk is also 3%. When one parent has clubfoot and has a child with clubfoot, the risk for clubfoot in additional children rises to 10 to 15%.

Although the disabling effects of clubfoot may often be prevented through early treatment, there is no method of totally preventing the defect at this time. Genetic counseling can help parents understand the odds with each pregnancy for having a child with clubfoot, as well as the outlook for treatment.

CYSTIC FIBROSIS

Cystic Fibrosis (CF) is a debilitating disease inherited from parents with autosomal recessive genes and results in the body producing abnormal amounts of thick, sticky mucus that clogs the lungs and pancreas, interfering with breathing and digestion. CF occurs in about one out of every fifteen hundred newborns and about an estimated 12 million Americans (one out of every 20) are unknowing carriers of the gene that causes CF. A child with the disorder must inherit a cystic fibrosis gene from each parent. Parents who have a cystic fibrosis child must both be carriers, and therefore, each additional child they conceive has a one in four chance of having the disease. For parents with a family history of cystic fibrosis, carrier detection and prenatal diagnosis is possible using DNA techniques.

Although there currently is no cure for cystic fibrosis, major advances have been made in recent years to minimize the rate of infection in CF patients, which has helped many extend their lives. Clinical trials with gene therapy are under way and may one day provide a cure for cystic fibrosis.

DUCHENNE MUSCULAR DYSTROPHY

This is an X-linked recessive disorder (affecting only males) with symptoms first appearing around the age of three or four. Symptoms include progressive wasting of the leg and pelvic muscles, followed by confinement to a wheelchair (usually by age 12) and heart disorders. Most boys with Duchenne muscular dystrophy die before the age of 20.

When a woman is a carrier, approximately 50% of her sons will develop Duchenne muscular dystrophy. Furthermore, about 50% of her daughters will be carriers, with the potential to pass the defective gene on to their sons. Unaffected sons of a female carrier cannot pass on the disease, because if they carried the gene for Duchenne muscular dystrophy, they would have it. Sometimes the disease occurs as a result of a new mutation in one of the reproductive cells that gave rise to the child. When this occurs, the mother of the affected son will not be the carrier and the chances of having future sons with the disorder is very rare.

There is no cure for muscular dystrophies. Continuous care from a team of health care providers, including physical, occupational, and respiratory therapists, helps individuals with muscular dystrophy maintain optimal muscle function and some degree of independence.

GALACTOSEMIA

This autosomal recessive disorder results in the body's inability to metabolize milk sugar. Two copies of the gene for galactosemia are required to produce the disease. If two normal parents have a child with galactosemia, both parents must be carriers for a galactosemia gene, and each additional child they produce will have a one in four chance of having the disease. If one parent has galactosemia, he or she will only produce children with galactosemia if the other parent is a carrier or also has the disease, both of which are unlikely unless the two parents are related. Therefore, few people with galactosemia give birth to children with the disorder. Prenatal diagnosis for galactosemia can be carried out on cells obtained through amniocentesis or chorionic villus sampling.

HEMOPHILIA

This inherited disorder characterized by excessive bleeding occurs almost exclusively in males. England's Queen Victoria, the daughter of Edward, Duke of Kent, was a carrier of this X-linked recessive gene, and it has shown up in many of her descendants. Because classic hemophilia results from an X-linked recessive gene, males must inherit only a single copy of the hemophilia gene to have the disease, as they possess only a single X chromosome. Females, on the other hand, must inherit two copies of the gene, one from each parent, to have the disease. That's why almost all classic hemophiliacs are male. Prenatal testing for hemophilia is now available for prospective parents.

HURLER'S SYNDROME

This autosomal recessive genetic disease occurs from the absence of an important enzyme that is needed for normal development. Infants born with this condition are born normal, but their condition deteriorates after one year of age, leading to a wide array of symptoms: enlargement of the head, liver and spleen; bone deformities; stunted growth; and mental retardation. Hurler's Syndrome is a rare disorder, occurring in approximately one in one hundred thousand births, and can be detected with prenatal diagnosis by amniocentesis.

MARFAN SYNDROME

This inherited abnormality (autosomal dominant disorder) is characterized by elongation of bones, especially the arms, legs, fingers, and toes; joint hypermobility and abnormality of the eyes (such as dislocation of the lens); and weakness in the aorta. It is suspected that Abraham Lincoln had this disorder, and more recently, 1984 U.S. Olympic volleyball team member Flo Hyman was diagnosed with Marfan syndrome when she died after her aorta ruptured during a volleyball match. Because Marfan syndrome is so rare, virtually all people with the disorder are heterozygous, which means they carry a single copy of the disease gene. Therefore, when one parent has Marfan syndrome, each child has a 50% chance of inheriting the disease.

PHENYLKETONURIA (PKU)

Today, all newborns are screened for this genetic disease. Early treatment can prevent its symptoms, which range all the way from poor muscle coordination and growth delay to severe mental retardation. More than any other disease, PKU illustrates the benefits of screening for genetic diseases. Because PKU is an autosomal recessive disease, a person with PKU will produce a PKU child only if their spouse also has the disorder or is a carrier for the PKU gene, both of which are very unlikely.

SICKLE CELL DISEASE (SICKLE CELL ANEMIA)

Sickle cell disease is one of the most common blood diseases. This autosomal recessive disorder is most common among people of African descent, occurring with a frequency of one out of every 625 births of African-Americans. It is estimated that as many as one in 12 African-Americans are carriers of the sickle cell gene. It also affects people of Arabian, Greek, Maltese, Italian, Scandinavian, Turkish, and Indian ancestry.

A child with sickle cell disease possesses two copies of the sickle cell gene—one inherited from each parent. When a couple has a child with sickle cell disease, each additional child they conceive has a one in four chance of having the disease. Carrier testing is available for detecting those individuals that carry the gene for sickle cell disease. Prenatal testing is also available and can be conducted through amniocentesis and chorionic villus sampling (CVS).

A few children with sickle cell disease have been cured through a bone marrow transplant, using donated bone marrow from an immunologically matched sibling. However, a cure using this approach carries a high risk. Other approaches that are being studied, such as gene therapy, may someday offer a cure at less risk.

THALASSEMIA

This autosomal recessive disorder occurs worldwide but is primarily seen in people of Mediterranean, Southeast Asian, Middle Eastern, or African descent. The disease encompasses a group of anemias in which a specific defect is present in the hemoglobin. Depending on whether the thalassemia mutation is inherited from one or both parents, there is an extreme variance in severity of symptoms. Thalassemia can be detected prenatally either through amniocentesis or chorionic villus sampling.

OTHER MEDICAL CONDITIONS WITH GENETIC LINKS

The following conditions are partly hereditary, so you may be at risk if one runs in your family, especially if it affects first-degree relatives (parents or siblings).

ALLERGIES

Researchers have always been puzzled by the occurrence of allergies. Genes have been linked, along with other factors, to allergic reactions. Most of us know firsthand that allergies tend to run in families. If you have hay fever, there's a good chance someone else in your family has it. In fact, about 50% of people who suffer from hay fever have other family members with hay fever. Most geneticists agree that allergies are multifactorial with the genes and the environment interacting to produce these conditions. Many researchers have also seen similar family histories of food allergies.

The best method to prevent allergic reactions is to avoid the specific allergen that triggers the attack. This, however, is not always possible or realistic. Medications can usually help control and relieve symptoms as well.

ARTHRITIS

Scientists have known for some time that people with certain genetic traits, or markers, are more likely than others to develop certain types of arthritis. Heredity appears to be involved in rheumatoid arthritis, but it does not follow any simple pattern of inheritance. A group of genes known as HLA-DR4 is associated with rheumatoid arthritis; however, some unaffected individuals also have these genes. This has led researchers to conclude that rheumatoid arthritis is an autoimmune disease.

ASTHMA

Recent research has shown a genetic connection to this respiratory disorder characterized by recurrent episodes of breathing difficulties. In some families, asthma appears to be inherited as an autosomal dominant trait; however, the inheritance appears to be more complicated in other families. Since asthma is often triggered by environmental factors (cold air, dust, pollen, animal hair, etc.), the genes involved must cause an underlying susceptibility, which is then expressed as the symptoms of asthma when the right environmental conditions are present. Therefore, most researchers concur that asthma is multifactorial in nature, resulting from an interaction of several genes and environmental factors.

BALDNESS

Researchers at Columbia University recently discovered the first human gene associated with balding. Male pattern (loss of hair from the front and top of the head) and premature balding are traits determined by a dominant gene on a nonsex chromosome (autosome). Although the gene can be present in males and females, it is usually expressed only in males because of the influence of male hormones. Females can carry the gene and pass it to offspring, but females rarely become bald; although with age their hair may thin dramatically.

MIGRAINE HEADACHES

The exact cause of migraine headaches is unknown, but they do run in families and occur more frequently in women.

Some people can identify certain factors such as specific foods, stress, or medications that trigger these excruciating headaches. Medication and behavior modification are generally recommended for preventing and treating migraine headaches.

OBESITY

Defined as being 20% or more over your ideal weight, obesity is known to increase your risk of heart disease, hypertension, diabetes, and some cancers. There is no single obesity gene, but if you notice that you gain weight easily, and others in your family are also heavy, genetic factors may be partially responsible. Statistics show that when both parents are obese, their children have an 80% chance of also being obese. However, when both parents have normal weight, the chance of their children being obese is less than 15%. How genes influence body weight is not clear. The genes affecting body weight may act on the basic metabolic rate of the body. In other words, some people may burn more calories in normal day-to-day activities than others, and these genetic differences in metabolic rate might affect differences in body weight.

If you're obese and haven't had any success with diet and exercise programs, your physician may prescribe a prescription drug that can help you lose weight by controlling appetite. However, because these medications have a wide range of side effects, it's extremely important that you are fully informed of the risks they may pose.

PERIODONTAL DISEASE (GUM DISEASE)

Dentists have known for a long time that periodontal disease, or gum disease, runs in families. It has been estimated that 100 million Americans suffer from periodontal disease to some degree. A recent study has also found that people infected with the bacteria that cause periodontal disease seem to be at double the risk of developing cardiovascular disease. The best way to prevent periodontal disease is to have regular dental checkups and practice good oral hygiene at home.

SPEECH DISORDERS

Just as this book was going to press, scientists located a single genetic defect on chromosome 7 that was responsible for a severe speech and language disorder. For some time, speech pathologists have pointed out that a variety of speech and language disorders tend to run in families. If you are concerned that your child has either a severe or mild speech disorder, discuss your concerns with your pediatrician, who may then refer your child to a speech therapist.

Appendix A: National Archives and Branches

MAIN ARCHIVES:

National Archives and
Records Administration
Pennsylvania Avenue at
8th Street, NW
Washington, DC 20408

REGIONAL BRANCHES:

National Archives
New England Region
380 Trapelo Road
Waltham, MA 02154
*—Serves Connecticut, Maine,
Massachusetts, New Hampshire,
Rhode Island, and Vermont.*

National Archives
Northeast Region
Building 22
Military Ocean Terminal
Bayonne, NJ 07002
*—Serves New Jersey, New York,
Puerto Rico, and the Virgin Islands.*

National Archives
Mid-Atlantic Region
9th and Market Streets
Room 1350
Philadelphia, PA 19107
*—Serves Delaware and Pennsylvania;
for microfilm loans also serves District
of Columbia, Maryland, Virginia,
and West Virginia.*

National Archives
Southeast Region
1557 St. Joseph Avenue
East Point, GA 30344
*—Serves Alabama, Florida, Georgia,
Kentucky, Mississippi, North Carolina,
South Carolina, and Tennessee.*

National Archives
Great Lakes Region
7358 South Pulaski Road
Chicago, IL 60629
*—Serves Illinois, Indiana, Michigan,
Minnesota, Ohio, and Wisconsin.*

National Archives
Central Plains Region
2312 East Bannister Road
Kansas City, MO 64131
*—Serves Iowa, Kansas, Missouri,
and Nebraska.*

National Archives
Southwest Region
501 West Felix Street
P.O. Building 6216
Forth Worth, TX 76115
—*Serves Arkansas, Louisiana, New Mexico, Oklahoma, and Texas.*

National Archives
Rocky Mountain Region
Building 48
Denver Federal Center
P.O. Box 25307
Denver, CO 80225
—*Serves Colorado, Montana, North Dakota, South Dakota, Utah, and Wyoming.*

National Archives
Pacific Sierra Region
1000 Commodore Drive
San Bruno, CA 94066
—*Serves California except southern California, Hawaii, Nevada except Clark County, and the Pacific Ocean area.*

National Archives
Pacific Southwest Region
24000 Avila Road
1st floor
P.O. Box 6719
Laguna Niguel, CA 92677
—*Serves Arizona; the southern California counties of Imperial, Inyo, Kern, Los Angeles, Orange, Riverside, San Bernardino, San Diego, San Luis Obispo, Santa Barbara, and Ventura; and Clark County, Nevada.*

National Archives
Pacific Northwest Region
6125 Sand Point Way NE
Seattle, WA 98115
—*Serves Idaho, Oregon, and Washington.*

National Archives
Alaska Region
654 West Third Avenue
Room 012
Anchorage, AK 99501
—*Serves Alaska only.*

Appendix B: Vital Records

Parenthetical notes indicate the date of the earliest record available at that particular location.

ALABAMA
(Marriage—1936; Birth and death—1908)
Center for Health Statistics
State Department of Public Health
434 Monroe Street
Montgomery, AL 36130
(205) 242-5033

ALASKA
(Marriage, birth, and death—1913)
Department of Health
Sciences and Social Services
Bureau of Vital Statistics
P.O. Box H-02G
Juneau, AK 99811
(907) 465-3392

AMERICAN SAMOA
Registrar of Vital Statistics
Vital Statistics Section
Government of American Samoa
Pago Pago, AS 96799

ARIZONA
(Marriage—Write to clerk of superior court in appropriate county; Birth and death—1909)
Vital Records Section
Arizona Department of
Health Services
P.O. Box 3887
Phoenix, AZ 85030
(602) 255-3260

ARKANSAS
(Marriage—1917; Birth and death—1914)
Division of Vital Records
Arkansas Department of Health
4815 West Markham St.
Little Rock, AR 72201
(501) 661-2336

CALIFORNIA
(Marriage, birth, and death—1905)
Vital Statistics Section
Department of Health Services
410 N. Street
P.O. Box 730241
Sacramento, CA 94244
(916) 445-2684

CANAL ZONE
Panama Canal Commission
Vital Statistics Clerk
APO Miami, FL 34011

COLORADO
*(Marriage, birth, and
death—1907)*
Vital Records Section
Colorado Department of Health
4210 East 11th Avenue
Denver, CO 80220
(303) 692-2227

CONNECTICUT
*(Marriage, birth, and
death—1897)*
Vital Records
Department of Health Services
150 Washington St.
Hartford, CT 06106
(203) 566-1124

DELAWARE
*(Marriage, birth, and
death—1930)*
Office of Vital Statistics
Division of Public Health
P.O. Box 637
Dover, DE 19903
(302) 739-4721

DISTRICT OF COLUMBIA
(Birth—1874; Death—1855)
Vital Records Branch
Room 3009
425 I Street, NW
Washington, DC 20001
(202) 727-9281

FLORIDA
*(Marriage—1927; Birth—1865;
Death—1877)*
Department of Health and
Rehabilitative Services
Office of Vital Statistics
1217 Pearl St.
P.O. Box 210
Jacksonville, FL 32202
(904) 359-6900

GEORGIA
*(Marriage—1952; Birth and
death—1919)*
Georgia Department of
Human Resources
Vital Records Unit
Room 217-H
47 Trinity Ave. SW
Atlanta, GA 30334
(404) 656-4750

GUAM
Office of Vital Statistics
Department of Public Health
Government of Guam
P.O. Box 2816
Agana, GU, M.I. 96910

HAWAII
(Marriage, birth, and death—1853)
Office of Health Status Monitoring
State Department of Health
P.O. Box 3378
Honolulu, HI 96801
(808) 961-7327

IDAHO

(Marriage—1947; Birth and death—1911)
Vital Statistics Unit
Idaho Department of
Health and Welfare
450 West State St.
Statehouse Mail
Boise, ID 83720
(208) 334-5988

ILLINOIS

(Marriage—1962; Birth and death—1916)
Division of Vital Records
Illinois Department of
Public Health
605 West Jefferson St.
Springfield, IL 62702
(217) 782-6553

INDIANA

(Marriage—1958; Birth—1907; Death—1900)
Vital Records Section
State Boards of Health
1330 West Michigan St.
P.O. Box 1964
Indianapolis, IN 46206
(317) 633-0276

IOWA

(Marriage, birth, and death—1880)
Iowa Department of Public Health
Vital Records Section
Lucas Office Building
321 East 12th St.
Des Moines, IA 50319
(515) 281-4944

KANSAS

(Marriage—1913; Birth and death—1911)
Office of Vital Statistics
Kansas State Department of
Health and Environment
900 Jackson St., SW
Topeka, KS 66612
(913) 296-1400

KENTUCKY

(Marriage—1958; Birth and death—1911)
Office of Vital Statistics
Department for Health Services
275 East Main St.
Frankfort, KY 40621
(606) 564-4212

LOUISIANA

(Marriage—1946; Birth and death—1914)
Vital Records Registry
Office of Public Health
325 Loyola Ave.
New Orleans, LA 70112
(504) 568-5152

(City of New Orleans only: Birth—1790; Death—1803)
Bureau of Vital Statistics
City of Health Department
City Hall
Civic Center
New Orleans, LA 70112

MAINE
(Marriage, birth, and death—1892)
Office of Vital Records
Human Services Building
Station 11
State House
Augusta, ME 04333
(207) 287-3181

MARYLAND
(Marriage—1951; Birth and death—1898)
Division of Vital Records
Department of Health and
Mental Hygiene
Metro Executive Building
4201 Patterson Ave.
P.O. Box 68760
Baltimore, MD 21215
(800) 832-3277

(City of Baltimore only: Birth and death—1875)
Bureau of Vital Statistics
Municipal Office Building
Baltimore, MD 21202

MASSACHUSETTS
(Marriage, birth, and death—1896)
Registry of Vital Records
and Statistics
150 Tremont St.
Room B-3
Boston, MA 02111
(617) 727-0036

(City of Boston only: Birth and death—1639)
City Registrar
Registry Division
Health Department
Room 705, City Hall Annex
Boston, MA 02133

MICHIGAN
(Marriage, birth, and death—1867)
Office of the State Registrar and
Center for Health Statistics
Michigan Department of
Public Health
3423 North Logan St.
Lansing, MI 48909
(517) 335-8656

MINNESOTA
(Marriage—1958; Birth and death—1908)
Minnesota Department of Health
Section of Vital Statistics
717 Delaware St. SE
P.O. Box 9441
Minneapolis, MN 55440
(612) 623-5121

MISSISSIPPI
(Marriage—1926; Birth and death—1912)
Vital Records
State Department of Health
2423 North State St.
Jackson, MS 39216
(601) 960-7981

MISSOURI

(Marriage—1948; Birth and death—1910)
Department of Health
Bureau of Vital Records
1730 East Elm St.
P.O. Box 570
Jefferson City, MO 65102
(314) 751-6400

MONTANA

(Marriage—1943; Birth and death—1907)
Bureau of Records and Statistics
State Department of Health and
Environmental Sciences
1400 Broadway
Box 200901
Helena, MT 59620
(406) 444-4228

NEBRASKA

(Marriage—1909; Birth and death—1904)
Bureau of Vital Statistics
State Department of Health
301 Centennial Mall South
P.O. Box 95007
Lincoln, NE 68509
(402) 471-2872

NEVADA

(Marriage—Write to county recorder of appropriate county; Birth and death—1911)
Division of Health-Vital Statistics
Capitol Complex
505 East King St., #102
Carson City, NV 89710
(702) 687-4480

NEW HAMPSHIRE

(Marriage, birth, and death—1640)
Bureau of Vital Records
Health and Human
Services Building
6 Hazen Dr.
Concord, NH 03301
(603) 271-4650

NEW JERSEY

(Marriage—Write to county recorder of appropriate county; Birth and death—1878)
State Department of Health
Bureau of Vital Statistics
South Warren and Market St.
CN 370
Trenton, NJ 08625
(609) 292-4087

NEW MEXICO

(Marriage—Write to county recorder of appropriate county; Birth and death—1880)
Vital Statistics
New Mexico
Health Services Division
1190 St. Francis Dr.
Santa Fe, NM 87503
(505) 827-2321

NEW YORK

(Marriage, birth, and death—1880)
Vital Records Section
State Department of Health
Empire State Plaza
Tower Building
Albany, NY 12237
(518) 474-3077

(New York City, Borough of Bronx, only: Marriage—1914; Birth and death—1898)
Bronx Bureau of Vital Records
1826 Arthur Ave.
Bronx, NY 10457

(New York City, Borough of Brooklyn, only: Marriage—1866; Birth and death—1898)
Brooklyn Bureau of Vital Records
Municipal Building
Brooklyn, NY 11201

(New York City, Borough of Manhattan, only: Marriage—1866; Birth and death—1898)
Bureau of Vital Records
Department of Health of
New York City
125 Worth St.
New York, NY 10016

(New York City, Borough of Queens, only: Marriage—1898)
Office of City Clerk
120-55 Queens Blvd.
Kew Gardens, NY 11424

(New York City, Borough of Queens, only: Birth and death—1898)
Queens Bureau of Vital Records
90-37 Parsons Blvd.
Jamaica, NY 11432

(New York City, Borough of Staten Island, only: Marriage—1898)
City Clerk's Office
Borough Hall
St. George
Staten Island, NY 10301

(New York City, Borough of Staten Island, only: Birth and death—1898)
Staten Island Bureau of
Vital Records
51 Stuyvesant Pl.
St. George
Staten Island, NY 10301

NORTH CAROLINA
(Marriage—1962; Birth and death—1913)
Department of Environment,
Health, and Natural Resources
Division of Epidemiology
Vital Records Section
P.O. Box 27687
Raleigh, NC 27611
(919) 733-3526

NORTH DAKOTA
(Marriage—1925; Birth and death—1893)
Division of Vital Records
State Capital
600 East Boulevard Ave.
Bismarck, ND 58505
(701) 224-2360

OHIO
(Marriage—1949; Birth and death—1908)
Division of Vital Statistics
Ohio Department of Health
P.O. Box 15098
Columbus, OH 43215
(614) 466-2531

OKLAHOMA
(Marriage—Write to clerk of appropriate county; Birth and death—1908)
Vital Records Section
State Department of Health 1000
Northeast 10th St.
P.O. Box 53551
Oklahoma City, OK 73152
(405) 271-4040

OREGON
(Marriage—1907; Birth and death—1903)
Oregon Health Division
Vital Statistics Section
P.O. Box 116
Portland, OR 97207
(503) 731-4095

PENNSYLVANIA
(Marriage—1941; Birth and death—1906)
Division of Vital Records
State Department of Health
Central Building
101 South Mercer St.
P.O. Box 1528
New Castle, PA 16103
(412) 656-3100

PUERTO RICO
Department of Health
Demographic Registry
P.O. Box 11854
Fernandez Juncos Station
San Juan, PR 00910

RHODE ISLAND
(Marriage, birth, and death—1853)
Division of Vital Records
Rhode Island
Department of Health
Room 101, Cannon Building
3 Capital Hill
Providence, RI 02908
(401) 277-2811

SOUTH CAROLINA
(Marriage—1950; Birth and death—1915)
Office of Vital Records and
Public Health Statistics
South Carolina
Department of Health and
Environmental Control
2600 Bull St.
Columbia, SC 29201
(803) 734-4830

SOUTH DAKOTA
(Marriage, birth, and death—1905)
State Department of Health
Center of Health Policy
and Statistics
Vital Records
523 East Capitol
Pierre, SD 57501
(605) 773-4961

TENNESSEE
(Marriage—1945; Birth and death—1914)
Tennessee Vital Records
Department of Health
and Environment
C3-324 Cordell Hull Building
Nashville, TN 37247
(615) 741-1763

*(City of Memphis, only: Birth—
1874; Death—1848)*
Shelby County
Health Department
Division of Vital Records
Memphis, TN 38105

TEXAS
*(Marriage—Write to county clerk
of appropriate county; Birth and
death—1903)*
Bureau of Vital Statistics
Texas Department of Health
1100 West 49th St.
Austin, TX 78756
(512) 458-7111

UTAH
*(Marriage—Write to county clerk
of appropriate county; Birth and
death—1905)*
Bureau of Vital Records
Utah Department of Health
288 North 1460 West
P.O. Box 16700
Salt Lake City, UT 84116
(801) 538-6105

VERMONT
*(Marriage—1857; Birth and
death—1760)*
Vermont Department of Health
Vital Records Section
60 Main Street
P.O. Box 70
Burlington, VT 05402
(802) 863-7275

VIRGINIA
(Marriage, birth, and death—1853)
Division of Vital Records
State Health Department
P.O. Box 1000
Richmond, VA 23208
(804) 786-6228

WASHINGTON
*(Marriage—1968; Birth and
death—1907)*
Vital Records
1112 South Quince
P.O. Box 9709, ET-11
Olympia, WA 98504
(206) 753-5936

WEST VIRGINIA
*(Marriage—1921; Birth and
death—1917)*
Vital Registration Office
Division of Health
State Capital Complex
Building 3
Charleston, WV 25305
(304) 348-2931

WISCONSIN
*(Marriage—1835; Birth and
death—1852)*
Vital Records
1 West Wilson St.
P.O. Box 309
Madison, WI 53701
(608) 266-1372

WYOMING
(Marriage—1941; Birth and death—1909)
Vital Records Services
Hathaway Building
Cheyenne, WY 82002
(307) 777-7591

Appendix C: Libraries with Excellent Genealogical Collections

ALABAMA
Alabama Genealogical Society
AGS Depository
and Headquarters
Samford University Library
800 Lakeshore Dr.
Birmingham, AL 35229

Birmingham Public Library
2100 Park Place
Birmingham, AL 35203

University of Alabama
William Stanley Hoole Special
Collections Library
Box 870266
Tuscaloosa, AL 35487-9784

ALASKA
Alaska Division of State Libraries
Pouch G
State Capitol
Juneau, AK 99801

Alaska State Library
Historical Collections
P.O. Box 110571
Juneau, AK 99811

University of Alaska, Fairbanks
College of Arts and Science
University of Alaska Museum
907 Yukon Drive
Fairbanks, AK 99701

ARIZONA
Arizona and the West Library
318 University of Arizona
Tucson, AZ 85721

Arizona Historical Society Library
949 East Second St.
Tucson, AZ 85719

Arizona State Department
of Library Archives and
Public Records
State Capital
1700 West Washington
Phoenix, AZ 85007

Flagstaff City Library
300 West Aspen
Flagstaff, AZ 86001

Tucson Public Library
200 S. 6th Ave.
Tucson, AZ 85701

ARKANSAS
Arkansas State Library
One Capital Mall
Little Rock, AR 72201

Little Rock Public Library
700 Louisiana St.
Little Rock, AR 72201

Pine Bluff and Jefferson
County Library
200 East 8th Ave.
Civic Center Complex
Pine Bluff, AR 71601

Southwest Arkansas
Regional Archives
Mary Medaris, Director
Old Washington Historic
State Park
Washington, AR 71862

CALIFORNIA
California State Archives
Rm. 200
1020 "0" St.
Sacramento, CA 95814

California State Library
California Section, Room 304
Library and Courts Building
914 Capitol Mall
Sacramento, CA 95814

California State Library
California Section
914 Capitol Mall
P.O. Box 942837
Sacramento, CA 94237

Genealogical Research Center
Department of Special Collections
San Francisco Public Library
480 Winston Drive
San Francisco, CA 94132

Huntington Library
1151 Oxford Rd.
San Marino, CA 91108

Long Beach Public Library
101 Pacific Ave.
Long Beach, CA 90822

Los Angeles Public Library
630 W. Fifth St.
Los Angeles, CA 90071

Oakland Public Library
125 14th St.
Oakland, CA 94612

Pasadena Public Library
285 E. Walnut
Pasadena, CA 91101

Pomona Public Library
P.O. Box 2271
Pomona, CA 91766

University of California, Berkeley
Bancroft Library
Berkeley, CA 94720

University of California
Los Angeles
Department of Special Collections
University Research Library
Floor A
Los Angeles, CA 90024-1575

COLORADO
Boulder Public Library
1000 Canyon Blvd.
Boulder, CO 80302

Colorado Historical Society
Stephen H. Hart Library
Colorado State History Museum
1300 Broadway
Denver, CO 80203

Colorado Springs Public Library
21 Kiowa St.
Colorado Springs, CO 80902

Denver Public Library
1357 Broadway
Denver, CO 80203

Historical Society Library
1300 Broadway
Denver, CO 80203

Montrose Public Library
434 South First
Denver, CO 81401

Norlin Library
University of Colorado
Campus Box 184
Boulder, CO 80309

Penrose Public Library
20 N. Cascade
Colorado Springs, CO 80902

Stagecoach Library
1840 S. Wolcott Ct.
Denver, CO 80219

Tutt Library
Special Collections
1021 North Cascade
Colorado Springs, CO 80903

CONNECTICUT
Connecticut Historical
Society Library
1 Elizabeth Street
Hartford, CT 06105

Connecticut State Library
231 Capitol Ave.
Hartford, CT 06115

Godfrey Memorial Library
134 Newfield St.
Middletown, CT 06457

Hartford Public Library
500 Main St.
Hartford, CT 06103

New Haven Public Library
133 Elm Street
New Haven, CT 06510

Otis Library
261 Main St.
Norwich, CT 06360

Public Library
63 Huntington St.
New London, CT 06320

Yale University Libraries
Box 1603A
Yale Station
New Haven, CT 06520

DELAWARE
Division of History
Department of State
Hall of Records
Dover, DE 19901

The Public Archives Commission
Hall of Records
Dover, DE 19901

University Library
University of Delaware
Newark, DE 19716

DISTRICT OF COLUMBIA
District of Columbia Public Library
Washingtoniana Division
901 G Street NW
Washington, DC 20001

Genealogical Department
Library of Congress Annex
Washington, DC 20540

Library of Congress
Local History and Genealogy
Reading Room Section
Thomas Jefferson Building
Room LJ244
101 Independence Avenue SE
Washington, DC 20540

National Archives and
Records Service
Washington, DC 20408

FLORIDA
Florida State Library
Supreme Court Bldg.
Tallahassee, FL 32304

Jacksonville Public Library
122 N. Ocean St.
Jacksonville, FL 32202

Miami-Dade Public Library
101 W. Flagler St.
Miami, FL 33130

Orlando Public Library
10 N. Rosalind Ave.
Orlando, FL 38201

Palm Beach County
Genealogical Library
Box 1746
W. Palm Beach, FL 33402

P.K. Yonge Library of
Florida History
University of Florida
404 Library West
Gainesville, FL 32611

State Library of Florida
R.A. Gray Bldg.
Tallahassee, FL 32301

Tampa Public Library
900 N. Ashley St.
Tampa, FL 33602

GEORGIA
Atlanta Public Library
1 Margaret Mitchell Sq.
Atlanta, GA 30303

Bradley Memorial Library
1120 Bradley Dr.
Columbus, GA 31995

Brunswick Regional Library
208 Gloucester St.
Brunswick, GA 31523

Carnegie Library
607 Broad St.
Rome, GA 30161

Decatur-DeKalb Library
215 Sycamore St.
Decatur, GA 30030

Genealogical Center Library
Box 71343
Marietta, GA 30007-1343

Georgia Department of
Archives and History
330 Capitol Ave.
Atlanta, GA 30334

Georgia Historical Society Library
501 Whittaker St.
Savannah, GA 31499

Georgia State Library
301 Judicial Bldg.
Capitol Hill Stn.
Atlanta, GA 30334

Georgia State University Archives
104 Decatur St. SE
Atlanta, GA 30303

Lake Lanier Regional Library
Pike St.
Lawrenceville, GA 30245

Piedmont Regional Library
189 Bellview St.
Winder, GA 30680

Savannah Public Library
2002 Bull St.
Savannah, GA 31401

Southwest Georgia
Regional Library
Shotwell at Monroe
Bainbridge, GA 31717

Washington Memorial Library
1180 Washington Ave.
Macon, GA 31201

HAWAII
Brigham Young University
Hawaii Campus
P.O. Box 1887
Laie, HI 96762

DAR Memorial Library
1914 Makiki Hts. Dr.
Honolulu, HI 96822

Library of Hawaii
King and Punchbowl Sts.
Honolulu, HI 96813

IDAHO
Boise State University Library
1910 University Dr.
Boise, ID 83725

Idaho Genealogical Library
450 North Fourth St.
Boise, ID 83702

Idaho State Historical Society
Library and Archives
450 North Fourth St.
Boise, ID 83702

Idaho State University Library
Pocatello, ID 83209

ILLINOIS
Chicago Historical Society
Research Collections
1601 N. Clark St.
Chicago, IL 60614

Illinois State Archives
Norton Bldg.
Springfield, IL 62706

Illinios State Historical Library
Old State Capitol
Springfield, IL 62756

Madison County Museum
and Library
715 N. Main St.
Edwardsville, IL 62025

Newberry Library
60 W. Walton St.
Chicago, IL 60610

Peoria Public Library
107 NE Monroe St.
Peoria, IL 61602

Rock Island Public Library
Rock Island, IL 61201

Rockford Public Library
215 N. Wyman St.
Rockford, IL 61101

University of Illinois
Library 346
1408 West Gregory Dr.
Urbana, IL 61801

Vogel Genealogical Library
305 North First St.
P.O. Box 132
Holcomb, IL 61043

INDIANA
Allen County Public Library
P.O. Box 2270
Fort Wayne, IN 46801

Genealogy Division
Indiana State Library
140 N. Senate St.
Indianapolis, IN 46204

Public Library of Fort Wayne
Ft. Wayne, IN 46802

IOWA
Iowa Genealogical Society Library
P.O. Box 7735
Des Moines, IA 50322

State Historical Society of
Iowa Library
402 Iowa Avenue
Iowa City, IA 52240

State Library of Iowa
East 12th and Grand
Des Moines, IA 50319

KANSAS
Bethel Historical Library
Kauffman Museum
Bethel College
North Newton, KS 67117

Garden City Public Library
605 East Walnut
Garden City, KS 67846

Johnson County Library
8700 W. 63rd St.
Shawnee Mission, KS 66201

Kansas State Historical
Society Library
Historical Research Center
120 West Tenth Street
Topeka, KS 66612

Public Library
220 East Maple St.
Independence, KS 67301

Public Library
6th and Minnesota St.
Kansas City, KS 66101

Topeka Public Library
1515 West 10th
Topeka, KS 66604

Wichita City Library
223 South Main Street
Wichita, KS 67202

KENTUCKY
Breckenridge County
Public Library
Hardinsburg, KY 40143

Kentucky Historical Society
KHS Library
Old Capital Annex
300 West Broadway
Box H
Frankfort, KY 40602-2108

Kentucky State Library
and Archives
Public Records Division
300 Coffee Tree Road
P.O. Box 537
Frankfurt, KY 40602-0537

Louisville Free Public Library
604 S. 10th St.
Louisville, KY 40203

National Society of the Sons of
the American Revolution
Genealogy Library
1000 South Fourth Street
Louisville, KY 40203

Western Kentucky
University Library
1 Big Red Way St.
Bowling Green, KY 42101

LOUISIANA
Hill Memorial Library
Louisiana State University
Baton Rouge, LA 70803

Howard Tilton Library
Map and Genealogy Room
Tulane University
6823 Saint Charles Ave.
New Orleans, LA 70118

Louisiana State Library
Box 131
Baton Rouge, LA 70821

New Orleans Public Library
219 Loyola Ave.
New Orleans, LA 70140

Quachita Parish Public Library
1800 Stubbs Ave.
Monroe, LA 71201

Shreve Memorial Library
424 Texas St.
Shreveport, LA 71120

Tangipahoa Parish Library
739 West Oak
Amite, LA 70422

MAINE
Bangor Public Library
145 Harlow St.
Bangor, ME 04401

Maine Historical Society Library
485 Congress Street
Portland, ME 04101

Maine State Library
State House
Augusta, ME 04330

MARYLAND
Enoch Pratt Free Library
400 Cathedral St.
Baltimore, MD 21201

George Peabody Library of
the John Hopkins University
17 E. Mt. Vernon Place
Baltimore, MD 21202

Hall of Records
Maryland State Archives
350 Rowe Boulevard
Annapolis, MD 21401

Maryland State Library
Court of Appeals Bldg.
361 Rowe Blvd.
Annapolis, MD 21401

MASSACHUSETTS
Boston Public Library
Box 286
Boston, MA 02117

Essex Institute
132 Essex St.
Salem, MA 01970

Massachusetts State Library
State House, Room 341
Beacon Street
Boston, MA 02133

New England Historic
Genealogical Society Library
101 Newbury Street
Boston, MA 02116

Secretary of the Commonwealth
Public Documents Division
State House
Boston, MA 02133

Springfield City Library
220 State Street
Springfield, MA 01103

MICHIGAN
Detroit Society for
Genealogical Research
Detroit Public Library
5201 Woodward Ave.
Detroit, MI 48202

Flint Public Library
1026 E. Kearsley
Flint, MI 48502

Grand Rapids Public Library
Michigan and Family
History Division
60 Library Plaza, NE
Grand Rapids, MI 49503

Herrick Public Library
300 River Ave.
Holland, MI 49423

Library of Michigan
717 W. Allegan
P.O. Box 30007
Lansing, MI 48909

Mason County Genealogical and
Historical Resource Center
c/o Rose Hawley Museum
305 E. Filer Street
Ludington, MI 49431

Michigan Department
of Education
State Library
Box 30007
Lansing, MI 48909

MINNESOTA
Folke Bernadette Memorial Library
Gustavus Adolphus College
800 W. College Ave.
St. Peter, MN 56082

Minneapolis Public Library
300 Nicollet Ave.
Minneapolis, MN 55401

Minnesota Historical Society
Library Reference Services
345 Kellogg Blvd., West
St. Paul, MN 55102

Public Library
90 W. 4th
St. Paul, MN 55102

Rolvaag Memorial Library
St. Olaf College
1510 Saint Olaf Ave.
Northfield, MN 55057

University of Minnesota Library
309 19th Ave. S
Minneapolis, MN 55455

MISSISSIPPI
Attala County Library
201 South Huntington Street
Kosciusko, MS 39090

Biloxi Public Library
P.O. Box 467
Biloxi, MS 39533

Department of Archives
and History
929 High Street
Jackson, MS 39202

Evans Memorial Library
105 North Long
Aberdeen, MS 39730

Lauren Rogers Memorial Library
Box 1108
Laurel, MS 39441

Mississippi State Department
of Archives and History
Archives and Library Division
100 South State Street
Box 571
Jackson, MS 39205

University of Mississippi Library
University, MS 38677

MISSOURI
Kansas City Public Library
311 E. 12th St.
Kansas City, MO 64106

Kent Library
Southeast Missouri State College
1 University Plz.
Cape Girardeau, MO 63701

Missouri Heritage Library
135 E. Pine St.
Warrenburg, MO 64093

Missouri Historical Society
Research Library
Jefferson Memorial Building
225 S. Skinker Blvd.
St. Louis, MO 63105

Missouri State Library
301 West High St.
P.O. Box 387
Jefferson City, MO 65102

Records and Archives
Office of Secretary of State
Capitol Bldg.
Jefferson City, MO 65101

Riverside Regional Library
Box 389
Jackson, MO 63755

St. Louis Public Library
1301 Olive St.
St. Louis, MO 63103

Springfield Public Library
Reference Department and
Shepard Room
397 E. Central St.
Springfield, MO 65801

MONTANA
Mansfield Library
University of Montana
Missoula, MT 59812

Montana Historical Society
Library/Archives
225 North Roberts
Helena, MT 59620

Montana State Library
1515 East Sixth Ave.
Helena, MT 59620

Parmly Billings Memorial Library
510 N. Broadway
Billings, MT 59101

Public Library
226 West Broadway
Butte, MT 59701

Public Library
301 East Maine
Missoula, MT 59802

State University Library
Missoula, MT 59801

NEBRASKA
Alliance Public Library
202 W. 4th St.
Alliance, NE 69301

Nebraska D.A.R. Library
202 W. 4th St.
Alliance, NE 69301

Nebraska State Historical
Society Library
1500 R St.
Box 82554
Lincoln, NE 68501

Omaha Public Library
215 S. 15th St.
Omaha, NE 68102

Public Library
136 S. 14th St.
Lincoln, NE 68508

University of Nebraska Library
Lincoln, NE 68588

Wayne Public Library
410 Main St.
Wayne, NE 68787

NEVADA
Las Vegas Public Library
400 E. Mesquite Ave.
Las Vegas, NV 89101

Nevada State Historical Society
1650 North Virginia Street
Reno, NV 89503

Nevada State Library and Archives
100 Stewart Street
Carson City, NV 89710

University of Nevada Library
Special Collections
University Library/322
Reno, NV 89557

Washoe County Library
629 Jones Street
Reno, NV 89503

NEW HAMPSHIRE
City Library
Carpenter Memorial Bldg.
405 Pine Street
Manchester, NH 03104

Dartmouth College Archives
Baker Memorial Library
Hanover, NH 03755

Dover Public Library
73 Locust St.
Dover, NH 03820

Exeter Public Library
10 Chestnut Street
Founders Park
Exeter, NH 03833

New Hampshire State Library
20 Park St.
Concord, NH 03301

NEW JERSEY
Atlantic City Free Library
1 North Tennessee Avenue
Atlantic City, NJ 08401

Morris Genealogical Library
228 Elberton Ave.
Allenhurst, NJ 07711

New Jersey Historical Society
230 Broadway
Newark, NJ 07104

New Jersey State Library
Archives and History Bureau
185 W. State St.
Trenton, NJ 08625

Rutgers University Library
169 College Ave.
New Brunswick, NJ 08901

NEW MEXICO
History Library Museum
of New Mexico
Palace of the Governors
Santa Fe, NM 87504

New Mexico State
Library Commission
325 Don Gasper Avenue
Santa Fe, NM 87503

New Mexico State Records
Center and Archives
404 Montezuma Street
Santa Fe, NM 87501

Public Library
423 Central Avenue, NE
Albuquerque, NM 87102

University of
New Mexico Library
Albuquerque, NM 87131

NEW YORK
Adriance Memorial Library
93 Market St.
Poughkeepsie, NY 12601

Buffalo and Erie County
Public Library
Lafayette Square
Buffalo, NY 14203

Columbia University
Journalism Library
New York, NY 10027

Flower Memorial Library
Genealogical Committee
229 Washington Street
Watertown, NY 13601

James T. Olin Library
Cornell University
201 Olin Library
Ithaca, NY 14853

New York Public Library
United States History, Local
History and Genealogy Division
5th Ave. and 42nd Sts.
Room 315N
New York, NY 10018

New York State Historical
Association Library
Lake Road
Box 800
Cooperstown, NY 13326

New York State Library
Genealogy Section
Seventh Floor, Cultural
Education Center
Empire State Plaza
Albany, NY 12230

New York-Ulster County
Elting Library
Historical and
Genealogical Department
93 Main Street
New Paltz, NY 12561

Queens Borough Public Library
8911 Merrick Blvd.
Jamaica, NY 11432

Rochester Public Library
Local History Division
115 South Avenue
Rochester, NY 14604

Roswell P. Flower
Genealogy Library
229 Washington St.
Watertown, NY 13601

Syracuse Public Library
335 Mongomery St.
Syracuse, NY 13202

NORTH CAROLINA
North Carolina State University
109 E. Jones Street
Raleigh, NC 27601

Public Library of Charlotte and
Mecklenburg Counties
310 N. Tryon St.
Charlotte, NC 28202

Rowan Public Library
201 W. Fisher St.
Salisbury, NC 28145

University of North Carolina,
Chapel Hill
CB 3930 Wilson Library
Chapel Hill, NC 27599-3930

NORTH DAKOTA
Public Library
102 North Third Street
Fargo, ND 58102

Public Library
2110 Library Circle
Grand Forks, ND 58201

Public Library
516 2nd Ave., SW
Minot, ND 58701

State Library
Liberty Memorial Building
Capital Grounds
Bismarck, ND 58505

University of North Dakota Library
P.O. Box 9000
Grand Forks, ND 58202

OHIO
Akron Public Library
55 South Main St.
Akron, OH 44326

American Jewish Archives
Hebrew Union College
3101 Clifton Ave.
Cincinnati, OH 45220

Cincinnati Public Library
800 Vine St.
Cincinnati, OH 45202

Cleveland Public Library
325 Superior Ave.
Cleveland, OH 44114

Dayton and Montgomery
Counties Public Library
215 E. 3rd St.
Dayton, OH 45402

Ohio Historical Society Library
1982 Velma Ave.
Columbus, OH 43211

Ohio State Library
65 South Front St.
Columbus, OH 43266

Portsmouth Public Library
1220 Gallia St.
Portsmouth, OH 45662

Public Library of Cincinnati and
Hamilton County
800 Vine St.
Cincinnati, OH 45202

Public Library of Columbus
96 S. Grant Ave.
Columbus, OH 43215

Public Library of Youngstown
305 Wick Ave.
Youngstown, OH 44503

Toledo Public Library
Historical and
Genealogical Department
325 Michigan St.
Toledo, OH 43624

University of Cincinnati
808 Blegen Library
Cincinnati, OH 45221

Warder Public Library
137 E. High St.
Springfield, OH 45502

Wayne County Public Library
304 N. Market St.
Wooster, OH 44691

OKLAHOMA
Carnegie Public Library
Carnegie, OK 73015-0009

Metropolitan Library System
131 Dean McGee Ave.
Oklahoma City, OK 73102

Oklahoma City Library
109 Capitol
Oklahoma City, OK 73105

Oklahoma State
Department of Libraries
200 NE 18th St.
Oklahoma City, OK 73105

Public Library
801 West Okmulgee
Muskogee, OK 74401

Public Library
220 S. Cheyenne
Tulsa, OK 74103

State D.A.R. Library
Historical Bldg.
Oklahoma City, OK 73105

Tulsa Central Library
400 Civic Center
Tulsa, OK 74103

University of Oklahoma
Western History Collections
630 Parrington Oval, Room 452
Norman, OK 73069

OREGON
Astoria Public Library
450 10th St.
Astoria, OR 97103

City Library
100 West 13th Avenue
Eugene, OR 97401

Oregon State Archives
Secretary of State
800 Summer Street, NE
Salem, OR 97310

Oregon State Library
State Library Bldg.
250 Winter St., NE
Salem, OR 97310

Portland Library Association
801 SW 10th Ave.
Portland, OR 97205

University of Oregon Library
1501 Kincaid St.
Eugene, OR 97401

PENNSYLVANIA
Altoona Public Library
"The Pennsylvania Room"
1600 5th Ave.
Altoona, PA 16602

Carnegia Library
4400 Forbes Ave.
Pittsburgh, PA 15213

Centre County Library
203 N. Allegheny St.
Bellefonte, PA 16823

Citizens Library
55 S. College St.
Washington, PA 15301

Fackenthall Library
Franklin and Marshall College
College Avenue and James Street
P.O. Box 3003
Lancaster, PA 17604

Franklin Institute Library
Benjamin Franklin Parkway
and 20th St.
Philadelphia, PA 19103

Free Library of Philadelphia
1901 Vine St.
Philadelphia, PA 19103

Friends Library
Swarthmore, PA 19081

Historical Society of
Pennsylvania Library
1400 Locust Street
Philadelphia, PA 19107

Lutheran Historical Society
Gettysburg, PA 17325

Lutheran Theological
Seminary Library
7301 Germantown Ave.
Philadelphia, PA 19119

Pennsylvania Historical and
Museum Commission
Division of Archives
Box 1026
Harrisburg, PA 17108

Pennsylvania State Library
Walnut and Commonwealth
Harrisburg, PA 17105

Reading Public Library
100 South Fifth Street
Reading, PA 19602

University Library
Pennsylvania State University
University Park, PA 16802

RHODE ISLAND
Providence Public Library
225 Washington St.
Providence, RI 02903

Rhode Island Historical
Society Library
110 Benevolent Street
Providence, RI 02906

Rhode Island State Archives
337 Westminster Street
Providence, RI 02903

Rhode Island State Library
Office of the Secretary of State
337 Westminster Street
Providence, RI 02903

SOUTH CAROLINA
Abbeville-Greenwood
Regional Library
N. Main St.
Greenwood, SC 29646

Free Library
404 King St.
Charleston, SC 29403

Greenville County Library
300 College St.
Greenville, SC 29601

Public Library
Rock Hill, SC 29730

Public Library
P.O. Box 2409
Spartanburg, SC 29304

Richland County Public Library
1431 Assembly Street #8
Columbia, SC 29201

South Carolina Archives
Department
1430 Senate St.
P.O. Box 11669
Columbia, SC 29211

South Carolina Library
University of South Carolina
301 Gervais St.
Columbia, SC 29201

South Carolina State Library
1500 Senate St.
Columbia, SC 29201

State Department of
Archives and History
Archives Search Room
Capitol Station, Box 11669
Columbia, SC 29211

SOUTH DAKOTA
Alexander Mitchell Public Library
519 South Kline St.
Aberdeen, SD 57401

Carnegie Free Public Library
10th and Dakota St.
Sioux Falls, SD 57102

South Dakota State
Historical Library
800 Governors Drive
Pierre, SD 57501-2294

University of South
Dakota Library
414 E. Clark St.
Vermillion, SD 57069

TENNESSEE
Chattanooga Hamilton County
Bicentennial Library
Genealogy/Local History
Department
1001 Broad St.
Chattanooga, TN 37402

Cossitt-Goodwyn Library
33 S. Front St.
Memphis, TN 38103

East Tennessee Historical Center
500 W. Church Ave.
Knoxville, TN 37902

Memphis Public Library
1850 Peabody
Memphis, TN 38104

Memphis State University Library
Mississippi Valley Collection
Memphis, TN 38104

Public Library of Knox County
McClung Historical Collection
600 Market St.
Knoxville, TN 37902

Public Library of Nashville and
Davidson County
225 Polk Avenue
Nashville, TN 37203

Tennessee State Library
and Archives
403 7th Ave. North
Nashville, TN 37243

TEXAS
Amarillo Public Library
300 East 4th
P.O. Box 2171
Amarillo, TX 79189

Catholic Archives to Texas
1600 Congress Ave.
Austin, TX 78801

Clayton Library for
Genealogical Research
5300 Caroline
Houston, TX 77004

Dallas Public Library
Genealogy Section
1515 Young Street
Dallas, TX 75201

El Paso Genealogical Library
3651 Douglas
El Paso, TX 79903

El Paso Public Library
501 N. Oregon St.
El Paso, TX 79901

Fort Worth Public Library
300 Taylor St.
Fort Worth, TX 76102

Genealogical Research Library
4524 Edmonson Ave.
Dallas, TX 75205

Houston Public Library
5300 Caroline Ave.
Houston, TX 77004

San Antonio Public Library
203 S. St. Mary's St.
San Antonio, TX 78205

Texarkana Public Library
600 West Third
Texarkana, TX 75501

Texas State Library
1201 Brazos St.
Austin, TX 78701

Waco Public Library
1717 Austin Ave.
Waco, TX 76701

UTAH
American Genealogical
Lending Library
Box 244
Bountiful, UT 84010

Brigham Carnegie Library
26 E. Forest
Brigham City, UT 84302

Brigham Young
University Library
Provo, UT 84602

Genealogical Library
Genealogical Society of
the Church of Jesus Christ of
Latter Day Saints
35 North West Temple
Salt Lake City, UT 84150

Logan Public Library
255 N. Main
Logan, UT 84321

Ogden Public Library
Ogden, UT 84402

University of Utah Library
Salt Lake City, UT 84112

Utah State Historical
Society Library
300 Rio Grande
Salt Lake City, UT 84101

Utah State University Library
Logan, UT 84321

VERMONT
Billings Library
Burlington, VT 05401

Genealogical Library
Bennington Museum
W. Main St.
Bennington, VT 05201

Public Library
10 Court St.
Rutland, VT 05701

The Russel Collection
c/o The Dorothy Canfield Library
Main Street
Arlington, VT 05250

University of Vermont Library
Burlington, VT 05401

Vermont Department of Libraries
Reference and Law Services
109 State St.
Montpelier, VT 05609

Vermont Historical
Society Library
Pavilion Office Bldg.
109 State St.
Montpelier, VT 05602

VIRGINIA
Albermarle County Historical
Library
220 Court Square
Charlottesville, VA 22901

Alderman Library
McCormick Rd.
Charlottesville, VA 22903

Alexandria Library
717 Queen St.
Alexandria, VA 22314

Commonwealth of Virginia
Virginia State Library
1101 Capitol
Richmond, VA 23219

E. Lee Trinkle Library
University of Virginia
Frederickson, VA 22402

Earl Gregg Swem Library
College of William and Mary
P.O. Box 8781
Williamsburg, VA 23187

Jones Memorial Library
2311 Memorial Ave.
Lynchburg, VA 24501

Kirn Norfolk Public Library
301 E. City Hall Ave.
Norfolk, VA 23510

Menno Simons Historical Library
Eastern Mennonite College
1200 Park Rd.
Harrisonburg, VA 22801

National Genealogical
Society Library
4527 Seventeenth Street, North
Arlington, VA 22207-2363

Virginia Historical Library
P.O. Box 7311
Richmond, VA 23211

Virginia State Library
11th St. at Capitol Square
Richmond, VA 23219-3491

WASHINGTON
Olympia Timberland Library
313 8th Ave., SE
Olympia, WA 98501

Public Library
P.O. Box 1197
Bellingham, WA 98225

Seattle Public Library
1000 4th Ave.
Seattle, WA 98104

Spokane Public Library
W. 906 Main Ave.
Spokane, WA 99201

University of Washington
Allen Library
Box 352900
Special Collections Division
Seattle, WA 98195

Washington State Historical
Society Library
State Historical Bldg.
315 North Stadium Way
Tacoma, WA 98403

Washington State Library
State Library Bldg.
Olympia, WA 98504-0111

WEST VIRGINIA
Cabell County Public Library
455 Ninth Street Plaza
Huntington, WV 25701

Morgantown Public Library
373 Spruce St.
Morgantown, WV 26505

State of West Virginia Library
Department of Archives and
Historical Library
Cultural Center
Capitol Complex
Charleston, WV 25305

West Virginia and Regional
History Collection
West Virginia University
Morgantown, WV 26502

WISCONSIN
Beloit Public Library
409 Pleasant St.
Beloit, WI 53511

Local History and
Genealogical Library
Racine County Historical Society
701 South Main Street
Racine, WI 53403

Milwaukee Public Library
814 W. Wisconsin Ave.
Milwaukee, WI 53233

State Historical Society
816 State Street
Madison, WI 53706-1482

University of Wisconsin
Milwaukee Library
P.O. Box 604
Milwaukee, WI 53211

WYOMING
American Heritage Department
University of Wyoming
Laramie, WY 82071

Wyoming State Archives
Museum and Historical
Department
Barrett Building
Cheyenne, WY 82002-0130

Wyoming State Library
Supreme Court and State
Library Building
Cheyenne, WY 82002

Appendix D: Genealogical and Historical Societies

ALABAMA
Alabama Genealogical Society
AGS Depository
Samford University Library
800 Lakeshore Dr.
Birmingham, AL 35229

Baldwin County
Genealogical Society
319 East Laurel Avenue
Foley, AL 36535

Birmington Genealogical Society
Box 2432
Birmingham, AL 35201

Butler County Historical Society
309 Fort Dale
Greenville, AL 36037

Civil War Descendants Society
P.O. Box 233
Athens, AL 35611

East Alabama
Genealogical Society
P.O. Box 2892
Opelika, AL 36803

Mobile Genealogical Society
Box 6224
Mobile, AL 36606

ALASKA
Anchorage Genealogy Society
Box 212265
Anchorage, AK 99521

Fairbanks, Alaska
Genealogical Society
P.O. Box 60534
Fairbanks, AK 99706

ARIZONA
Arizona Genealogical Society
6521 East Fayette St.
Tucson, AZ 85730-2220

Arizona Jewish Historical Society
4181 E. Pontatoc Canyon Dr.
Tucson, AZ 85718

Arizona State Genealogical Society
Box 42075
Tucson, AZ 85733-2075

Genealogical Society of Arizona
P.O. Box 27237
Tempe, AZ 85282

Phoenix Genealogical Society
6220 North 35th Drive
Phoenix, AZ 85019

ARKANSAS
Arkansas Genealogical Society
P.O. Box 908
Hot Springs, AR 71902

Faulkner County Historical Society
Conway, AR 72032

Hempstead County
Historical Society
P.O. Box 1158
Hope, AR 71801

Madison County
Genealogical Society
P.O. Box 427
Huntsville, AR 72740

Northeast Arkansas
Genealogical Association
314 Vine Street
Newport, AR 73112

Northwest Arkansas
Genealogical Society
P.O. Box 796
Rogers, AR 72757

Pulaski County Historical Society
P.O. Box 653
Little Rock, AR 72203

CALIFORNIA
California Genealogical Society
P.O. Box 77105
San Francisco, CA 94107-0105

Contra Costa County
Genealogical Society
Box 910
Concord, CA 94522

Fresno Genealogical Society
Box 1429
Fresno, CA 93716

Genealogical Society of Riverside
Box 2557
Riverside, CA 92516

Genealogical Society of
Santa Cruz County
Box 72
Santa Cruz, CA 95063

Hi Desert Genealogical Society
P.O. Box 1271
Victorville, CA 92392

Historical Society of
Southern California
200 E. Ave. 43
Los Angeles, CA 90031

Jewish Genealogical
Society of Los Angeles
4530 Woodley Ave.
Encino, CA 91436

Jewish Genealogical
Society of San Diego
255 South Rios Ave.
Solana Beach, CA 92075

Kern County Genealogical Society
Box 2214
Bakersfield, CA 93303

Los Angeles Westside
Genealogical Society
P.O. Box 10447
Marina del Rey, CA 90295

Mendicino County
Historical Society
603 West Perkins Street
Ukiah, CA 95482

Orange County
Genealogical Society
711 Talbert Avenue
Huntington Beach, CA 92648

Paradise Genealogical Society
Box 460
Paradise, CA 95969-0460

Redwood Genealogical Society
Box 645
Fortuna, CA 95540

San Bernardino Valley
Genealogical Society
P.O. Box 2220
San Bernardino, CA 92406

San Diego Genealogical Society
2925 Kalinna Street
San Diego, CA 92104

San Francisco Bay Area Jewish
Genealogical Society
40 West 3rd Ave.
San Mateo, CA 94402

San Mateo County
Historical Association
P.O. Box 5083
San Mateo, CA 94402

Sonoma County
Genealogical Society
P.O. Box 2273
Santa Rosa, CA 95405

Southern California
Genealogical Society
P.O. Box 4477
Burbank, CA 91503

Sutter-Yuba Genealogical Society
Box 1274
Yuba City, CA 95991

COLORADO
Boulder Genealogical Society
Box 3246
Boulder, CO 80303

Colorado Genealogical Society
P.O. Box 9218
Denver, CO 80209

Colorado Historical Society
Colorado Heritage Center
1300 Broadway
Denver, CO 80203

Eastern Colorado Historical Society
43433 Road CC
Cheyenne Wells, CO 80810

Larimer County
Genealogical Society
P.O. Box 9502
Fort Collins, CO 80524

Mesa County Genealogical Society
P.O. Box 1506
Grand Junction, CO 81502

CONNECTICUT
Brookfield, Connecticut
Historical Society
44 Hopbrook Rd.
Brookfield, CT 06804

Connecticut Genealogical Society
P.O. Box 435
Glastonburg, CT 06033

Connecticut Historical Society
1 Elizabeth St.
Hartford, CT 06105

Jewish Genealogical
Society of Connecticut
25 Soneham Rd.
West Hartford, CT 06117

New Haven Colony
Historical Society
114 Whitney Ave.
New Haven, CT 06510

Stamford Genealogical Society
Box 249
Stamford, CT 06904

DELAWARE
Delaware Genealogical Society
505 Market Street Mall
Wilmington, DE 19801

Delaware Society, Sons of the
American Revolution
P.O. Box 2169
Wilmington, DE 19899

Division of Historical and
Cultural Affairs
Department of State
Hall of Records
Dover, DE 19901

DISTRICT OF COLUMBIA
Afro-American Historical and
Genealogical Society
Box 73086
Washington, DC 20009-3086

National Society of the Children
of the American Revolution
1776 D Street NW
Washington, DC 20006

National Society of the Colonial
Dames of the XVII Century
1300 New Hampshire Ave., NW
Washington, DC 20036

National Society of the Daughters
of the American Revolution
1776 D Street NW
Washington, DC 20006-5392

Society of the Cincinnati
2118 Massachusetts Avenue, NW
Washington, DC 20008

White House Historical
Association
740 Jackson Place, NW
Washington, DC 20506

FLORIDA
Florida Genealogical Society
P.O. Box 18642
Tampa, FL 33609

Genealogical Society of
Greater Miami
P.O. Box 162905
Miami, FL 33116-2905

Hillsborough Bounty
Historical Commission
Museum Historical and
Genealogical Library
County Courthouse
Tampa, FL 33602

Jewish Genealogical
Society of Central Florida
P.O. Box 520583
Longwood, FL 32752

Manasota Genealogical
Society, Inc.
1405 4th Ave. West
Bradenton, FL 34205

Palm Beach County
Genealogical Society
Box 1746
W. Palm Beach, FL 33402

Polk County Genealogical Society
Box 1719
Bartow, FL 33830

Polk County
Historical Association
P.O. Box 2749
Bartow, FL 33830-2749

Southern Genealogist's
Exchange Society
Box 2801
Jacksonville, FL 32203

GEORGIA
Central Georgia
Genealogical Society
P.O. Box 2024
Warner Robbins, GA 31093

Chattahoochee Valley
Historical Society
1213 Fifth Avenue
West Point, GA 31833

Georgia Genealogical Society
Box 54575
Atlanta, GA 30308

Northeast Georgia Historical and
Genealogical Society
127 North Main
Gainesville, GA 30501

HAWAII
Hawaii Society, Sons of
the American Revolution
1564 Pikea St.
Honolulu, HI 96818

Hawaiian Historical Society
560 Kawaiahao St.
Honolulu, HI 96813

IDAHO
Idaho Genealogical Society
4620 Overland Road #204
Boise, ID 83705

Idaho Historical Society
325 State St.
Boise, ID 83702

Nez Perce Historical Society
P.O. Box 86
Nez Perce, ID 83542

ILLINOIS
Bloomington-Normal
Genealogical Society
Box 488
Normal, IL 61761-0488

Chicago Genealogical Society
P.O. Box 1160
Chicago, IL 60690

Chicago Historical Society
1601 N. Clark St.
Chicago, IL 60614

Cumberland and Coles County
Genealogical Society
1816 Walnut
Mattoon, IL 61938

Decatur Genealogical Society
Box 1548
Decatur, IL 62526

Genealogical Society of
Southern Illinois
c/o Logan College
Carterville, IL 62918

Great River Genealogical Society
c/o Quincy Public Library
526 Jersey St.
Quincy, IL 62301

Illiana Genealogical Society
Box 207
Danville, IL 61832

Illinois State Genealogical Society
P.O. Box 10195
Springfield, IL 62791

Iroquois County
Genealogical Society
Old Courthouse Museum
103 W. Cherry St.
Watseka, IL 60970

Jewish Genealogical
Society of Illinois
818 Mansfield Court
Schaumburg, IL 60194

Knox County Genealogical Society
Box 13
Galesburg, IL 61402-0013

Lexington Genealogical Society
318 West Main St.
Lexington, IL 61753

Moultrie County
Genealogical Society
Box 588
Sullivan, IL 61951

Peoria Genealogical Society
Box 1489
Peoria, IL 61655

Peoria Historical Society
942 N.E. Glen Oak Ave.
Peoria, IL 61600

Sangamon County
Genealogical Society
Box 1829
Springfield, IL 62705

INDIANA
Delaware County
Historical Alliance
P.O. Box 1266
Muncie, IN 47308

Elkhart County
Genealogical Society
1812 Jeanwood Drive
Elkhart, IN 46514

Genealogical Section of the
Indiana Historical Society
140 N. Senate Ave.
Indianapolis, IN 46204

Indiana Genealogical Society
P.O. Box 10507
Fort Wayne, IN 46852

Indiana Historical Society
315 W. Ohio Street
Indianapolis, IN 46202

Marion County Historical Society
140 N. Senate
Indianapolis, IN 46204

Pulaski County
Genealogical Society
121 South Riverside Drive
Winamac, IN 46996

IOWA
Des Moines County
Genealogical Society
P.O. Box 493
Burlington, IA 52601

Iowa Genealogical Society
Box 7735
Des Moines, IA 50322

Lee County Genealogical Society
Box 303
Keokuk, IA 52632

State Historical Society of Iowa
600 E. Locust
Des Moines, IA 50319

KANSAS
Douglas County Historical Society
Watkins Community Museum
1047 Massachusetts St.
Lawrence, KS 66044

Finney County
Genealogical Society
P.O. Box 592
Garden City, KS 67846

Forsyth Library
600 Park Street
Room 122
Hays, KS 67601

Heritage Genealogical Society
502 Indiana Ave.
Neodesha, KS 66757

Johnson County
Genealogical Society
P.O. Box 12666
Shawnee Mission, KS 66282

Kansas Genealogical Society
Memorial Bldg.
Topeka, KS 66603

Montgomery County
Genealogical Society
Box 444
Coffeyville, KS 67337

Osborne County Genealogical
and Historical Society
Osborne Public Library
325 W. Main
Osborne, KS 67473

Riley County Genealogical Society
2005 Claflin Road
Manhattan, KS 66502

Topeka Genealogical Society
P.O. Box 4048
Topeka, KS 66604-0048

KENTUCKY
Central Kentucky
Genealogical Society
Box 153
Frankfort, KY 40601

Jewish Genealogical
Society of Louisville
Annette and Milton Russman
3304 Furman Blvd.
Louisville, KY 40220

Kentucky Genealogical Society
P.O. Box 153
Frankfort, KY 40602

Kentucky Historical Society
P.O. Box H
Frankfort, KY 40205

West-Central Kentucky Family
Research Association
P.O. Box 1932
Owensboro, KY 42302

LOUISIANA
Ark-La-Tex Genealogical
Assn., Inc.
P.O. Box 4462
Shreveport, LA 71134

Central Louisiana
Genealogical Society
P.O. Box 12206
Alexandria, LA 71315-2006

Genealogical Research
Society of New Orleans
P.O. Box 51791
New Orleans, LA 70150

Louisiana Genealogical and
Historical Society
Box 3454
Baton Rouge, LA 70821

North Louisiana
Genealogical Society
509 West Alabama
Ruston, LA 71270

MAINE
Maine Genealogical Society
P.O. Box 221
Farmington, ME 04938

Maine Historical Society
485 Congress St.
Portland, ME 04111

Old York Historical Society
P.O. Box 312
York, ME 03909

MARYLAND
Allegany County Historical Society
218 Washington St.
Cumberland, MD 21502

Genealogical Club of
the Montgomery County
Historical Society
103 W. Montgomery Ave.
Rockville, MD 20850

Jewish Historical
Society of Maryland
15 Lloyd St.
Baltimore, MD 21202

Maryland Genealogical Society
201 West Monument St.
Baltimore, MD 21201

MASSACHUSETTS
American Jewish Historical Society
2 Thorton Rd.
Waltham, MA 02154

Massachusetts Historical Society
1154 Boylston St.
Boston, MA 02215

New England Historic and
Genealogical Society
101 Newberry St.
Boston, MA 02116

Winchester Historical Society
1 Copley Street
Winchester, MA 01890

MICHIGAN
Detroit Society for
Genealogical Research
Detroit Public Library
5201 Woodward Ave.
Detroit, MI 48202

Flint Genealogical Society
P.O. Box 1217
Flint, MI 48501

Genealogical Association of
Southwestern Michigan
Box 573
St. Joseph, MI 49085

Jewish Genealogical
Society of Michigan
4987 Bantry Drive
West Bloomfield, MI 48322

Kalamazoo Valley
Genealogical Society
P.O. Box 405
Kalamazoo, MI 49041

Michigan Genealogical Council
Box 80953
Lansing, MI 48908

Michigan Historical Commission
505 State Office Bldg.
Lansing, MI 48913

Mid-Michigan
Genealogical Society
Box 16033
Lansing, MI 48901

Muskegon County
Genealogical Society
Hackley Library
316 W. Webster Ave.
Muskegon, MI 49440

Saginaw Genealogical Society
c/o Saginaw Public Library
505 Janes Ave.
Saginaw, MI 48507

Western Michigan
Genealogical Society
Grand Rapids Public Library
60 Library Plz., NE
Grand Rapids, MI 49503

MINNESOTA
Anoka County
Genealogical Society
1900 3rd Ave.
Anoka, MN 55303

Minnesota Genealogical Society
P.O. Box 16069
St. Paul, MN 55116

Minnesota Historical Society
690 Cedar St.
St. Paul, MN 55101

Range Genealogical Society
Box 388
Chisolm, MN 55719

MISSISSIPPI
Mississippi Genealogical Society
P.O. Box 5301
Jackson, MS 39216

Northeast Mississippi Historical
and Genealogical Society
P.O. Box 434
Tupeol, MS 38801

Vicksburg Genealogical Society
P.O. Box 1161
Vicksburg, MS 39181

MISSOURI
The Heart of America
Genealogical Society
c/o Missouri Valley Rm.
Kansas City Public Library
311 E. 21st St.
Kansas City, MO 64106

Missouri Genealogical Society
P.O. Box 382
St. Joseph, MO 64502

Missouri Historical Society
Jefferson Memorial Building
225 S. Skinker Blvd.
St. Louis, MO 63105-2317

Missouri State
Genealogical Association
P.O. Box 833
Columbia, MO 65205-0833

Ozarks Genealogical Society
Box 3494
Springfield, MO 64804

St. Louis Genealogical Society
9011 Manchester Road #3
St. Louis, MO 63144

The State Historical
Society of Missouri
1020 Lowry Street
Columbia, MO 65201

West Central Missouri
Genealogical Society
P.O. Box 435
Warrensburg, MO 64093

MONTANA
Lewis and Clark County
Genealogical Society
P.O. Box 5313
Helena, MT 59604

Montana Historical Society
225 N. Roberts St.
Helena, MT 59620

Montana State
Genealogical Society
P.O. Box 555
Chester, MT 59522

NEBRASKA
Fort Kearny Genealogical Society
P.O. Box 22
Kearny, NE 68847

Greater Omaha
Genealogical Society
P.O. Box 4011
Omaha, NE 68104

Madison County
Genealogical Society
P.O. Box 1031
Norfolk, NE 68702

Nebraska State
Genealogical Society
P.O. Box 5608
North Platte, NE 68505

North Platte Genealogical Society
P.O. Box 1452
North Platte, NE 69101

NEVADA
Clark County, Nevada
Genealogical Society
P.O. Box 1929
Las Vegas, NV 89125-1929

Jewish Genealogical
Society of Las Vegas
P.O. Box 29342
Las Vegas, NV 89126

Nevada State Genealogical Society
P.O. Box 20666
Reno, NV 89515

NEW HAMPSHIRE
Historical Society of
Cheshire County
P.O. Box 803
Keene, NH 03431

New Hampshire Historical
Society Library
30 Park Street
Concord, NH 03301

New Hampshire
Society of Genealogists
Strafford County Chapter
P.O. Box 633
Exeter, NH 03833

NEW JERSEY
Genealogical Society of New Jersey
P.O. Box 1291
New Brunswick, NJ 08903

Jewish Genealogical
Society of North Jersey
1 Bedford Road
Pompton Lakes, NJ 07442

New Jersey Historical Society
230 Broadway
Newark, NJ 07014

NEW MEXICO
New Mexico Genealogical Society
P.O. Box 8283
Albuquerque, NM 87198-8330

New Mexico Jewish
Historical Society
1428 Miracerros South
Santa Fe, NM 87501

Southern New Mexico
Genealogical Society
1017 Ivydale Drive
Las Cruces, NM 88005

NEW YORK
Albany Jewish
Genealogical Society
Rabbi Don Cashman
P.O. Box 3850
Albany, NY 12203

Brooklyn Historical Society
128 Pierrepont St.
Brooklyn, NY 11201

Central New York
Genealogical Society
P.O. Box 104
Colvin Station
Syracuse, NY 13205

Colonial Dames of America
421 East 61st Street
New York, NY 10021

General Society of Colonial Wars
122 East 58th St.
New York, NY 10022

Jewish Genealogical Society
P.O. Box 6398
New York, NY 10128

National Society of Colonial
Dames of America in the
State of New York Library
215 East 71st Street
New York, NY 10021

New York Genealogical and
Biographical Society
122-126 East 58th Street
New York, NY 10022

New York State
Historical Association
Fenimore House
Lake Rd.
Cooperstown, NY 13326

Suffolk County Historical Society
300 W. Main St.
Riverhead, NY 11901

Twin Tiers Genealogical Society
P.O. Box 763
Elmira, NY 14902

Ulster County Genealogical Society
P.O. Box 536
Hurley, NY 12443

NORTH CAROLINA

Alleghany Historical-Genealogical
Society
P.O. Box 817
Sparta, NC 28675

Genealogical Society of the
Original Wilkes County
North Wilkesboro, NC 28659

Jewish Genealogy Society
of Raleigh
8701 Sleepy Creek Dr.
Raleigh, NC 27612

North Carolina
Genealogical Society
P.O. Box 1492
Raleigh, NC 27602

North Carolina Society of
County and Local Historians
1209 Hill St.
Greensboro, NC 27408

NORTH DAKOTA

Bismarck-Mandan
Genealogical Society
P.O. Box 485
Bismarck, ND 58540

McLean County
Genealogical Society
P.O. Box 51
Garrison, ND 58540

Mouse River Loop
Genealogy Society
Box 1391
Minot, ND 58702-1391

State Historical Society of
North Dakota
Liberty Memorial Bldg.
Bismarck, ND 58501

OHIO

Ashtabula County
Genealogical Society
Henderson Library
54 East Jefferson Street
Jefferson, OH 44047

Cincinnati Historical Society
1301 Western Ave.
Cincinnati, OH 45203-1129

Genealogical Society
Morley Public Library
184 Phelps Street
Parinsville, OH 44077

Hardin County Historical Society
P.O. Box 503
Kenton, OH 43326

Jewish Genealogical
Society of Cleveland
996 Eastlawn Dr.
Highland Heights, OH 44143

Miami Valley Genealogical Society
P.O. Box 1364
Dayton, OH 45401

Northwestern Ohio
Genealogical Society
P.O. Box 17066
Toledo, OH 43615

Ohio Genealogical Society
P.O. Box 2625
Mansfield, OH 44906

Wayne County Historical Society
546 E. Bowman Street
Wooster, OH 44691

West Augusta Genealogical Society
1510 Prairie Dr.
Belpre, OH 45714

OKLAHOMA
Federation of Oklahoma
Genealogical Societies
P.O. Box 26151
Oklahoma City, OK 73126

Love County Historical Society
P.O. Box 134
Marietta, OK 73448

Oklahoma Genealogical Society
Box 12986
Oklahoma City, OK 73101

Tulsa Genealogical Society
Box 585
Tulsa, OK 74157

OREGON
ALSI Historical and Genealogical
Society, Inc.
P.O. Box 822
Waldport, OR 97394

Coos Bay Genealogical Forum
Box 1067
Coos Bay, OR 97459

Genealogical Forum of Portland
1410 SW Morrison, Rm. 812
Portland, OR 97205

Jewish Genealogical
Society of Oregon
7335 SW Linette Way
Beaverton, OR 97007

Klamath Basin
Genealogical Society
1555 Hope St.
Klamath Falls, OR 97603

Mt. Hood Genealogical Forum
Box 744
Oregon City, OR 97045

Oregon Genealogical Society
P.O. Box 10306
Eugene, OR 97440-2306

Rogue Valley Genealogical Society
133 South Central Ave.
Medford, OR 97501

Williamette Valley
Genealogical Society
P.O. Box 2083
Salem, OR 97308

PENNSYLVANIA

Adams County Pennsylvania
Historical Society
P.O. Box 4325
Gettysburg, PA 17325

Bucks County
Genealogical Society
P.O. Box 1092
Doylestown, PA 18901

Erie County Historical Society
117 State St.
Erie, PA 16501

Erie Society for
Genealogical Research
P.O. Box 1403
Erie, PA 16512

Genealogical Society of
Pennsylvania
1300 Locust Street
Philadelphia, PA 19107

Genealogical Society of
Southwestern Pennsylvania
P.O. Box 894
Washington, PA 15301

Historical Society of
Berks County
940 Centre Ave.
Reading, PA 19601

Historical Society of
Montgomery County
1654 DeKalb St.
Norristown, PA 19401

Jewish Genealogical
Society of Philadelphia
332 Harrison Ave.
Elkins Park, PA 19117

Pennsylvania German Society
Box 97
Breinigsville, PA 18031

Presbyterian Historical Society
425 Lombard St.
Philadelphia, PA 19147

Somerset County Historical and
Genealogical Society
Road 2
Box 238
Somerset, PA 15501

South Central Pennsylvania
Genealogical Society
P.O. Box 1824
York, PA 17405

RHODE ISLAND

Newport Historical Society
82 Touro St.
Newport, RI 02840

Rhode Island
Genealogical Society
13 Countryside Drive
Warwick, RI 02864

Rhode Island State
Historical Society
52 Power St.
Providence, RI 02906

SOUTH CAROLINA

South Carolina Genealogical
Association
P.O. Box 1442
Lexington, SC 29072

South Carolina Historical Society
P.O. Box 5401
Spartanburg, SC 29304

SOUTH DAKOTA

Rapid City Society for
Genealogical Research
Box 1495
Rapid City, SD 57701

South Dakota
Genealogical Society
Route 2, Box 10
Burke, SD 57523

Tri-State Genealogical Society
905 5th St.
Belle Fourche, SD 57717

TENNESSEE

East Tennessee Historical Society
314 W. Clinch Ave.
Knoxville, TN 37902-2505

Mid-West Tennessee
Genealogical Society
P.O. Box 3343
Jackson, TN 38301

Morgan County Genealogical
and Historical Society
P.O. Box 684
Wartburg, TN 37887

Tennessee Genealogical Society
P.O. Box 111249
Memphis, TN 38111-1249

Watauga Association
of Genealogists
P.O. Box 117
Johnson City, TN 37605-0117

TEXAS

Amarillo Genealogical Society
Amarillo Public Library
413 East Fourth Street
P.O. Box 2171
Amarillo, TX 79189

Austin Genealogical Society
P.O. Box 1507
Austin, TX 78767-1507

Central Texas
Genealogical Society
1717 Austin Ave.
Waco, TX 76701

Chaparral Genealogical Society
P.O. Box 606
Tomball, TX 77375

Dallas Genealogical Society
P.O. Box 12648
Dallas, TX 75225

East End Historical Association
P.O. Box 2424
Galveston, TX 77550

East Texas Genealogical Society
P.O. Box 6967
Tyler, TX 75711

El Paso Genealogical Society
El Paso Main Public Library
501 N. Oregon Street
El Paso, TX 79901

Fort Worth Genealogical Society
P.O. Box 9767
Ft. Worth, TX 76107

Hispanic Genealogical Society
P.O. Box 810561
Houston, TX 77281-0561

Houston Area
Genealogical Association
2507 Tannehill
Houston, TX 77008-3052

Jewish Genealogical
Society of Houston
P.O. Box 980126
Houston, TX 77098

McLennan County Society
1717 Austin Ave.
Waco, TX 76701

Mesquite Genealogical Society
Box 850165
Mesquite, TX 75185

Methodist Historical Society
Southern Methodist University
Fondren Library
Box 750135
Dallas, TX 75275-0135

San Antonio Genealogical Society
P.O. Box 17461
San Antonio, TX 78217-0461

Southeast Texas
Genealogical Society
c/o Tyrell Historical Library
P.O. Box 3827
Beaumont, TX 77701

Tip O'Texas Genealogical Society
410 76 Drive
Harlingen, TX 78550

UTAH
Genealogical Society of Utah
35 North West Temple
Salt Lake City, UT 84150

Jewish Genealogical
Society of Salt Lake City
3510 Fleetwood Drive
Salt Lake City, UT 84109

St. George Genealogy Club
P.O. Box 184
St. George, UT 84770

Utah Genealogical Association
P.O. Box 1144
Salt Lake City, UT 84110

VERMONT
Burlington, Vermont
Genealogical Group
36 Franklin Square
Burlington, VT 05401

Genealogical Society of Vermont
P.O. Box 422
Pittsford, VT 05763

Vermont Historical Society
Pavillion Office Building
109 State Street
Montpelier, VT 05602

VIRGINIA
American Society of Genealogists
2255 Cedar Lane
Vienna, VA 22180

Central Virginia
Genealogical Association
P.O. Box 5583
Charlottesville, VA 22905

Fairfax Historical Society
P.O. Box 415
Fairfax, VA 22030

Genealogical Research
Institute of Virginia
P.O. Box 29178
Richmond, VA 23229

Genealogical Society of Tidewater
P.O. Box 76
Hampton, VA 23669

Jewish Genealogy Society of
Greater Washington
P.O. Box 412
Vienna, VA 22180

National Genealogical Society
4527 17th St. North
Arlington, VA 22207-2363

WASHINGTON
Eastern Washington
Genealogical Society
Box 1826
Spokane, WA 99210

Lower Columbia
Genealogical Society
Box 472
Longview, WA 98632

North Central Washington
Genealogical Society
P.O. Box 5280
Wenatchee, WA 98807

Olympia Genealogical Society
Box 1313
Olympia, WA 98507

Puget Sound Genealogical Society
P.O. Box 601
Tracyton, WA 98393-0601

Seattle Genealogical Society
Box 1708
Seattle, WA 98111

The Tacoma Genealogical Society
P.O. Box 1952
Tacoma, WA 98401

Tri-City Genealogical Society
P.O. Box 1410
Richland, WA 99352-1410

Washington State
Genealogical Society
Box 1422
Olympia, WA 98507

Washington State Historical
Society Library
State Historical Building
315 North Stadium Way
Tacoma, WA 98403

Whatcom County Washington
Genealogical Society
P.O. Box 1493
Bellingham, WA 98227-1493

WEST VIRGINIA
Marion County
Genealogical Club
321 Monroe Street
Fairmont, WV 26554

West Virginia
Genealogical Society
P.O. Box 249
Elkview, WV 25071

West Virginia Historical Society
Cultural Center
Capitol Complex
Charleston, WV 25305

Wetzel County
Genealogical Society
Box 464
New Martinsville, WV 26155

WISCONSIN
Jewish Genealogical Society
of Milwaukee
9280 N. Fairway Dr.
Milwaukee, WI 53217

Milwaukee County
Genealogical Society
P.O. Box 27326
Milwaukee, WI 53202

State Historical
Society of Wisconsin
University of Wisconsin
816 State St.
Madison, WI 53217

Wisconsin State
Genealogical Society
2109 20th Avenue
Monroe, WI 53566

WYOMING
Cheyenne Genealogical Society
2800 Central Ave.
Cheyenne, WY 82001

Converse County
Genealogical Society
119 N. 9th St.
Douglas, WY 82633

Appendix E: National Genetic Volunteer Organizations

Acoustic Neuroma
Association (ANA)
P.O. Box 12402
Atlanta, GA 30355
(404) 237-8023
—*Support and information for those who face or have undergone acoustic neuroma removal and those experiencing cranial nerve defects.*

Alliance of Genetics
Support Groups
35 Wisconsin Circle, Suite 440
Chevy Chase, MD 20815-7015
(800) 336-GENE

Alzheimer's Association
919 N. Michigan Avenue
Suite 1000
Chicago, IL 60611
(800) 272-3900
website: www.alz.org

American Brain Tumor
Association (ABTA)
2720 River Road, Suite 146
Des Plaines, IL 60018
(800) 886-2282
website: www.ABTA.org

American Cancer Society, Inc.
1599 Clifton Road, NE
Atlanta, GA 30329
(800) ACS-2345
website: www.cancer.org
—*Has more than three thousand local units.*

American Cleft
Palate-Craniofacial
Association (ACPA)
1218 Grandview Avenue
Pittsburgh, PA 15211
(412) 481-1376

American Diabetes Association
1660 Duke Street
Alexandria, VA 22314
(800) ADA-DISC
website: www.diabetes.org
—*Has seven hundred chapters in all 50 states and the District of Columbia.*

American Foundation for the
Blind, Inc. (AFB)
15 West 16th Street
New York, NY 10011

American Heart Association
7272 Greenville Avenue
Dallas, TX 75231
(800) 242-8721
website: www.amhrt.org

American Liver Foundation
1425 Pompton Avenue
Cedar Grove, NJ 07009
(800) 223-0179
website: http://gi.ucsf.edu/alf

American Lung Association
1740 Broadway
New York, NY 10019
(800) LUNG-USA
website: www.lungusa.org

American Lupus Society
3914 Del Amo Boulevard, #922
Torrance, CA 90503
(800) 331-1802

American Parkinson's
Disease Association
60 Bay Street, Suite 401
Staten Island, NY 10301
(800) 223-APDA

American Porphyria Foundation
P.O. Box 22712
Houston, TX 77227
(713) 266-9617
—Deals with group of rare blood
disorders.

American Tuberous Sclerosis
Association, Inc. (ATSA)
P.O. Box 44
Rockland, MA 02370

Amyotrophic Lateral Association
21021 Ventura Boulevard
Suite 321
Woodland Hills, CA 91364
(800) 782-4747
website: www.alsa.org

Arthritis Foundation
1330 W. Peachtree Street
Atlanta, GA 30309
(800) 886-2282
website: www.arthritis.org.

Association for Children with
Down's Syndrome, Inc.
2616 Martin Avenue
Bellmore, NY 11701

Association for Glycogen
Storage Disease
Box 896
Durant, IA 52747
(319) 785-6038

Association for Macular
Disease, Inc.
210 East 64th Street
New York, NY 10021
(212) 605-3719

Association for
Neuro-Metabolic Disorders
5223 Brookfield Lane
Sylvania, OH 43560
(419) 885-1497
—Serves those affected with medical conditions caused by disturbances in body chemistry.

Caring, Inc.
P.O. Box 400
Milton, WA 98354
—*Provides various support materials for parents and professionals interested in health and welfare of persons with Down's syndrome.*

Celiac-Sprue Association
(CSA/USA)
P.O. Box 31700
Omaha, NE 68131
(402) 558-0600
—*Provides material and dietary information about celiac-sprue and the gluten-free diet.*

Charcot-Marie-Tooth Association
c/o Crozer Mills Entpr. Center
601 Upland Avenue
Upland, PA 19015
(215) 499-7486
—*Helps those with CMT syndrome, also known as peroneal muscular atrophy, and provides a registry for researchers, enabling them to locate individuals for analyses.*

Children and Adults with
Attention Deficit Disorders
499 NW 70th Avenue, Suite 101
Plantation, FL 33317
(954) 587-3700
website: www.chadd.org

Coalition for Heritable
Disorders of Connective Tissue
382 Main Street
Port Washington, NY 11050
(800) 862-7326

Cooley's Anemia Foundation, Inc.
129-09 26th Avenue
Flushing, NY 11354
(800) 221-3571

Cornelia de Lange Syndrome
(CdLS) Foundation, Inc.
60 Dyer Avenue
Collinsville, CT 06022
(800) 223-8355

Cystic Fibrosis (CF) Foundation
6931 Arlington Road
Bethesda, MD 20814
(800) FIGHT-CF
website: www.ccf.org

Cystinosis Foundation, Inc.
1212 Broadway, #830
Oakland, CA 94612
(510) 235-1052

The Dysautonomia Foundation
20 E. 46th Street, 3rd floor
New York, NY 10017
(212) 949-6644

Dystonia Medical
Research Foundation
1 East Wacker, Suite 2900
Chicago, IL 60601
(312) 755-0198

Dystrophic Epidermolysis Bullosa
Research Association of America,
Inc. (D.E.B.R.A)
Kings County Medical Center
451 Clarkson Avenue Building
6th Floor, Room E6101
Brooklyn, NY 11203

Ehlers Danlos National Foundation
6399 Wilshire Blvd., #510
Los Angeles, CA 90048-5708
—*This foundation is interested in collecting family history records.*

Epilepsy Foundation of America
4351 Garden City Drive
Landover, MD 20785
(800) 332-1000
website: www.efa.org

Familial Polyposis Registry
Department of Colorectal Surgery
Cleveland Clinic Foundation
Building A-111
9500 Euclid Avenue
Cleveland, OH 44106

Families of S.M.A.
(Spinal Muscular Atrophy)
P.O. Box 1465
Highland Park, IL 60035
(800) 458-8655
—*Promotes public awareness of Werdnig-Hoffman disease, Kugelberg-Welander disease, benign congenital hypotonia, and Aran-Duchenne disease.*

The Foundation Fighting Blindness
Executive Plaza 1, Suite 800
11350 McCormick Road
Hunt Valley, MD 21031
(410) 785-1414
website: www.blindness.org

Friedreich's Ataxia Group in
America, Inc.
P.O. Box 11116
Oakland, CA 94611
—*A primary goal is to benefit persons with Friedreich's ataxia and their families.*

Glaucoma Research Foundation
490 Post Street, Suite 830
San Francisco, CA 94102
(415) 986-3162
website: www.glaucoma.org

The Gluten Intolerance Group
of North America (GIG)
P.O. Box 23053
Seattle, WA 98102-0353
—*Offers assistance and information to persons with celiac-sprue and to their families through publications and seminars and by funding research.*

Guardians of Hydrocephalus
Research Foundation
2618 Avenue Z
Brooklyn, NY 11235
(800) 458-8655

The Hemochromatosis Research Foundation, Inc.
P.O. Box 8569
Albany, NY 12208
(518) 489-0972
—*Hemochromatosis is one of the most common genetic disorders (a disorder of iron metabolism in which iron accumulates in tissues) but is rarely diagnosed before clinically manifest or before death. The organ damage that results from the disease is reversible and preventable with early diagnosis and treatment. One of the Foundation's goals is to identify families with the disorder through screening.*

Hereditary Disease Foundation
1427 7th Street, Suite 2
Santa Monica, CA 90401
(310) 458-4183

The Huntington's Disease Society of America, Inc. (HDSA)
140 West 22nd Street, 6th Floor
New York, NY 10011
(800) 345-4372
website: www.hdsa.mgh.harvaRoadedu/

Hydrocephalus Parent Support Group
225 Dickenson Street, H-893
San Diego, CA 92130
—*Deals with issues when a child is affected with hydrocephalus, spina bifida, or a related condition. Social interaction between families is encouraged.*

International Institute for Visually Impaired, 0-7, Inc.
1975 Rutgers
East Lansing, MI 48823
—*For preschool visually impaired children.*

International Joseph Diseases Foundation, Inc. (IJDF)
P.O. Box 2550
Livermore, CA 94550
(510) 443-4600
—*Services to those affected by, or at risk of inheriting, Joseph disease.*

International Rett's Syndrome Association (IRSA)
9121 Piscataway Road, #2B
Clinton, MD 20735
(301) 856-3334

Iron Overload Diseases Association, Inc. (IOD)
433 Westwind Drive
North Palm Beach, FL 33408
(407) 840-8512

Juvenile Diabetes Foundation (JDF) International
120 Wall Street, 19th floor
New York, NY 10005
(212) 785-9500
website: www.jdfcure.com

Susan G. Komen Breast Cancer Foundation
5005 LBJ, Suite 370
Dallas, TX 75244
(800) IM-AWARE

Laurence-Moon-Bardet-Biedl
Syndrome (LMBS)
Support Network
18 Strawberry Hill
Windsor, CT 06095
(203) 688-7880

Leukemia Society of America, Inc.
600 Third Avenue, 4th floor
New York, NY 10016
(800) 955-4LSA
website: www.leukemia.org

The Lupus Foundation of
America, Inc.
1300 Piccard Drive, Suite 200
Rockville, MD 20850
(301) 670-9292
website: www.lupus.org/lupus

Malignant Hyperthermia
Association of the United
States (MHAUS)
32 S. Main St.
Sherburne, NY 13460

March of Dimes Birth
Defects Foundation
1275 Mamaroneck Avenue
White Plains, NY 10605
(914) 428-7100
website: www.modimes.org

Melanoma Research Foundation
P.O. Box 747
San Leandro, CA 94577
(800) MRF-1290
website: www.melanoma.org

Mothers United for Moral
Support (MUMS)
150 Custer Court
Green Bay, WI 54301
(414) 336-5333

Multiple Sclerosis Foundation
6350 N. Andrews Avenue
Ft. Lauderdale, FL 33309
(800) 441-7055
website: www.msfacts.org

Muscular Dystrophy
Association (MDA)
3300 E. Sunrise Drive
Tucson, AZ 85718
(800) 572-1717
website: www.mdausa.org

Myasthenia Gravis Foundation,
Inc. (MGF)
222 S. Riverside Plaza
Suite 1540
Chicago, IL 60606
(800) 541-5454
website: www.med.unc.edu/mgfa/

National Association for the
Craniofacially Handicapped
P.O. Box 11082
Chattanooga, TN 37401

The National Association
for Parents of the Visually
Impaired, Inc. (NAPVI)
P.O. Box 180806
Austin, TX 78718

National Association for Sickle
Cell Disease, Inc. (NASCD)
3345 Wilshire Boulevard
Suite 1106
Los Angeles, CA 90010-3503
(800) 421-8453

National Association for
Visually Handicapped
305 East 24th Street, 17-C
New York, NY 10010

National Association of the Deaf
814 Thayer Avenue
Silver Spring, MD 20910
(301) 587-1788

National Ataxia Foundation
750 Twelve Oaks Center
15500 Wayzata Boulevard, #750
Wayzata, MN 55391
(612) 473-7666
*—Hereditary spastic paraplegia,
ataxia telangiectasia, and Charcot-
Marie-Tooth syndrome.*

National Center for Study
of Wilson's Disease
432 W. 58th Street, #614
New York, NY 10019
(212) 523-8717

National Down's Syndrome Society
141 Fifth Avenue, Suite 75
New York, NY 10010

National Easter Seal Society
230 W. Monroe Street
Suite 1800
Chicago, IL
(312) 726-6200
website: www.seals.com

National Foundation for
Ectodermal Dysplasias (NFED)
219 E. Main
Box 114
Mascoutah, IL 62258
(618) 566-2020

The National Foundation for
Jewish Genetic Diseases
250 Park Avenue, Suite 1000
New York, NY 10017
(212) 371-1030
*—Genetic diseases affecting descen-
dants of Eastern and Central
European Jews: familial dysautonomia, torsion dystonia, Gaucher's
disease, and mucolipidosis IV.*

National Fragile X Foundation
1441 York Street, #215
Denver, CO 80206
(800) 688-8765

National Gaucher
Foundation (NGF)
19241 Montgomery Village
Avenue, E-21
Gaithersburg, MD 20879
(301) 990-3800

The National Hemophilia
Foundation (NHF)
The Soho Building
110 Greene Street, Room 303
New York, NY 10002
(212) 219-8180
website: www.infonhf.org

The National Hydrocephalus
Foundation (NHF)
400 N. Michigan Avenue, #1102
Chicago, IL 60611
(815) 467-6548

National Kidney
Cancer Association
1234 Sherman Avenue, Suite 203
Evanston, IL 60202
(847) 332-1051
website: www.nkca.org

National Kidney Foundation, Inc.
2 Park Avenue
New York, NY 10016

National Marfan Foundation
54 Irma Avenue
Port Washington, NY 11050

National Multiple Sclerosis Society
733 Third Avenue, 6th floor
New York, NY 10017
(800) 344-4867
website: www.nmss.org

The National Neurofibromatosis
Foundation, Inc. (NF)
95 Pine Street, 16th floor
New York, NY 10005
(212) 344-NNFF
website: www.nf.org

National Organization for
Albinism and Hypopigmentation
(NOAH)
1500 Locust Street, Suite 2405
Philadelphia, PA 19102
(800) 473-2310

National Organization for Rare
Disorders, Inc. (NORD)
P.O. Box 8923
New Fairfield, CT 06812
(800) 999-NORD

National Osteoporosis Foundation
1150 17th Street, NW, Suite 500
Washington, DC 20036
(202) 223-2226
website: www.nof.org

National Ovarian Cancer Coalition
1451 W. Cypress Creek Road
#300
Fort Lauderdale, FL 33309
(954) 351-9555
website: www.ovarian.org

National Scoliosis Foundation, Inc.
P.O. Box 547
93 Concord Avenue
Belmont, MA 02178

National Society for Children
and Adults with Autism
1234 Massachusetts Avenue, NW
Suite 1017
Washington, DC 20005-4599

The National Tay-Sachs and
Allied Diseases Association, Inc.
(NTSAD)
2001 Beacon Street
Brookline, MA 02146
(617) 277-4463

National Tuberous Sclerosis
Association, Inc. (NTSA)
8181 Professional Place, #110
Landover, MD 20785
(800) 225-6872
website: www.ntsa.org

The Organic Acidemia Association
c/o Carol Breton
2287 Cypress Avenue
San Pablo, CA 94806
(510) 724-0297
—*Deals with organic acidemias
and related rare metabolic disorders.*

Orton Dyslexia Society
Chester Building, Suite 382
8600 LaSalle Road
Baltimore, MD 21286
(800) ABCD-123

Paget Foundation for Paget's Disease
of Bone and Related Disorders
120 Wall Street, Suite 1602
New York, NY 10005
(800) 23P-AGET
website: www.healthanswers.com/
health_answers/nhc/index.htm

Parkinson's Disease Foundation
William Black Medical
Research Building
Columbia-Presbyterian
Medical Center
640-650 West 168th Street
New York, NY 10032
(800) 457-6676

Prader-Willi Syndrome
Association (PWSA)
2510 S. Brentwood, #220
Saint Louis, MO 63144
(800) 926-4797

Prevent Blindness America
500 East Remington Road
Schaumburg, IL 60173
(847) 843-2020
website: www.prevent-blindness.org

The Scoliosis Association, Inc.
P.O. Box 811705
Boca Raton, FL 33481
(800) 800-0669

Sickle Cell Disease
Association of America
200 Corporate Pointe, Suite 495
Culver City, CA 90230
(800) 421-8453

Spina Bifida Association
of America (SBAA)
4590 MacArthur Boulevard, NW
Suite 250
Washington, DC 20007
(202) 944-3285
website: www.sbaa.org

Support Organization for Trisony
18/13 (SOFT)
c/o Barb VanHeireweghe
2982 S. Union Street
Rochester, NY 14624
(716) 594-4621

Tourette Syndrome
Association, Inc. (TSA)
42-40 Bell Boulevard
Bayside, NY 11361
(800) 237-0717
website: tsa.mgh.harvaRoadedu/

Turner's Syndrome Society
c/o Georgia Tesch
5500 Wayzata Boulevard
#768-214
Wayzata, MN 55391
(800) 365-9944

United Cerebral Palsy
Associations, Inc. (UCPA)
66 E. 34th Street
New York, NY 10016

United Leukodystrophy
Foundation, Inc. (ULF)
2304 Highland Drive
Sycamore, IL 60178
(800) 728-5483

United Parkinson's
Foundation (UPF)
833 W. Washington Boulevard
Chicago, IL 60607
(312) 733-1893

Wilson's Disease Association
P.O. Box 75324
Washington, DC 20013
—*For Wilson's or Menkes disease.*

Xeroderma Pigmentosum Registry
c/o Dept. of Pathology
Room C-520
Medical Science Building
UMDNJ-New Jersey
Medical School
100 Bergen Street
Newark, NJ 07103

Books Available From Santa Monica Press

The Book of Good Habits
Simple and Creative Ways to Enrich Your Life
BY DIRK MATHISON
224 pages $9.95

Collecting Sins
A Novel
BY STEVEN SOBEL
288 pages $13

Health Care Handbook
A Consumer's Guide to the American
Health Care System
BY MARK CROMER
256 pages $12.95

Helpful Household Hints
BY JUNE KING
224 pages $12.95

How to Find Your Family Roots
The Complete Guide to Searching for Your
Ancestors
BY WILLIAM LATHAM
224 pages $12.95

How to Win Lotteries, Sweepstakes, and Contests
BY STEVE LEDOUX
224 pages $12.95

Letter Writing Made Easy!
Featuring Sample Letters for Hundreds of
Common Occasions
BY MARGARET MCCARTHY
224 pages $12.95

Letter Writing Made Easy!
Volume 2
Featuring More Sample Letters for Hundreds of
Common Occasions
BY MARGARET MCCARTHY
224 pages $12.95

Offbeat Golf
A Swingin' Guide to a Worldwide Obsession
BY BOB LOEFFELBEIN
192 pages $17.95

Offbeat Marijuana
The Life & Times of the
World's Grooviest Plant
BY SAUL RUBIN
240 pages $19.95

Offbeat Museums
The Curators and Collections of America's Most
Unusual Museums
BY SAUL RUBIN
240 pages $17.95

Past Imperfect: How Tracing Your Family Medical History Can Save Your Life
BY CAROL DAUS
240 pages $12.95

What's Buggin' You?
Michael Bohdan's Guide to Home Pest Control
BY MICHAEL BOHDAN
256 pages $12.95

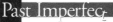

Order Form
1-800-784-9553

	Quantity	Amount
THE BOOK OF GOOD HABITS ($9.95)		
COLLECTING SINS ($13)		
HEALTH CARE HANDBOOK ($12.95)		
HELPFUL HOUSEHOLD HINTS ($12.95)		
HOW TO FIND YOUR FAMILY ROOTS ($12.95)		
HOW TO WIN LOTTERIES, SWEEPSTAKES . . . ($12.95)		
LETTER WRITING MADE EASY! ($12.95)		
LETTER WRITING MADE EASY! VOLUME 2 ($12.95)		
OFFBEAT GOLF ($17.95)		
OFFBEAT MARIJUANA ($19.95)		
OFFBEAT MUSEUMS ($17.95)		
PAST IMPERFECT: HOW TRACING YOUR FAMILY MEDICAL HISTORY CAN SAVE YOUR LIFE ($12.95)		
WHAT'S BUGGIN' YOU? ($12.95)		

Shipping & Handling:

1 book $3.00
Each additional book is $ .50

Subtotal _____

Shipping and Handling (see left) _____

CA residents add 8.25% sales tax _____

TOTAL _____

Name _____

Address _____

City_____ State _____ Zip _____

❏ Visa   ❏ MasterCard   Card Number_____

Signature _____

❏ Enclosed is my check or money order payable to:

Santa Monica Press LLC
P.O. Box 1076
Santa Monica, CA 90406
www.santamonicapress.com
smpress@pacificnet.net

1-800-784-9553